# 8 Keys To Longevity After 50

## Simple Habits And Ways To Live A Longer And Better Life

**Dr. Chio Ugochukwu**

# 8 Keys To Longevity  After  50

**Disclaimer**

The information contained in this book is based on research and the personal and professional experience of the author. It is solely for informational and educational purposes and should not be regarded as a substitute for professional, legal, tax, psychological or medical advice. Any attempt to diagnose or treat an illness should be done under the care of a healthcare professional. The author and publisher do not advocate any healthcare protocol but believe the information in this book should be available to the public. Ideas on ways people can get more peace and happiness in their relationships and their lives are shared in this book. The author assumes no liability or responsibility for any adverse effects or consequences from the use of any information, idea or instruction contained in this book.

**Dedication**

This book is dedicated to all those who want simple habits and ways to live a healthier and longer life. Are you ready to begin your own 30-day challenge for a longer life today? Age is not a barrier!

# 8 Keys To Longevity  After  50

## Table of Contents

"Your present circumstances
don't determine
where you can go;
they merely determine
where you start."

Nido Qubein

# 8 Keys To Longevity After 50

## Introduction

Do you want to stay healthy, active, independent, and live a more fulfilled life as you get older, or do you want to spend your time unintentionally going from one clinic and hospital to another being treated from one illness to another?

If you want to be able to hang out with your friends, go on vacations, participate in your friends' milestones or your kids and grandkids milestones like graduations, birthdays, weddings and other festivals and events that you enjoy doing as you get older then read this book to learn the 8 keys to longevity after 50.

Do you know the 8 keys that can help you live longer after 50? Do you know the commonest causes of death or chronic health conditions for those 50 and above? Do you know the most common health problems in your family or family history?

# 8 Keys To Longevity After 50

Did you know that by changing how you think about yourself, your situation and circumstances and deciding to take daily focused positive action, you can develop healthy lifestyles that will help you live a healthier, longer, and more fulfilled life? Through this book I will share with you the steps and actions that will help you protect your health and take good care of yourself as you get older.

You will learn how to live a healthier, more positive, less stressful, and longer life as you get older. You will also learn practical and easy ways to make adjustments that will help you improve your self-care and increase your peace of mind and joy of living as you get older. You will learn how to live the telomeric lifestyle!

Did you know that the first key to living longer after 50 is consistency in your daily exercise and physical activity? Don't live in denial or form the habit of always having reasons or excuses for not doing your daily exercise. Don't forget that the transformation that you need is within your power.

You can challenge yourself to use the 8 keys to longevity after 50,  that I will share with you in this book to transform your health and your life in 30 days or less and become a more positive, less stressed, healthier  and more fulfilled version of yourself.

Through this book you will learn the simple habits and  changes you can make in your lifestyle, eating habits or your relationships that can help you improve your health from the cellular and vascular level, through your organs to your mind, body and spirit, so that you can live a healthier, longer, and more holistic fulfilled life as you get older. You will begin to live the best telomeric lifestyle!

# 8 Keys To Longevity  After  50

## Form the habit of consistently doing more physical activity every day

Do you know that forming the habit of exercising and doing more physical activity every day is the first key to living a healthier and longer life? Research has shown that people as old as 69 years and above who exercise regularly  have the heart, lung, and muscle fitness of healthy people as young as 30 years and  younger (Crouch, 2019). Wouldn't you like to feel much younger than your age as you get older?

If you want to feel much younger than your age, make out time from your busy schedule to exercise more every day. Begin by doing your own 72 -hour health and wellness audit or simply walking log or fitness audit to find out how many minutes in a day you are physically active. This will help you know where you are in your longevity journey and what you need to do to become better.

Unfortunately, according to the National Institute of Health, only about 30 percent of people  between 45 years and 64 years engage in leisure-time physical activity, and for those 65 years above the percentage drops to 15 percent and less ( NIH News, 2017). According to the AARP, only about 17 % of Americans 50 years and above, do at least 150 minutes of exercise every week. Are you among those who exercise or among those who do not? What is the cellular link between exercise and physical activity and antiaging and living longer? It is telomere or specific-DNA structures found at both ends of our chromosomes.

According to Bringham Young University researchers, exercise has antiaging effects at the cellular level because increasing physical activity increased the length of telomeres at the end of chromosomes which are usually shorter with age. The study also found that those who exercise  had a "biological age" that was about nine years younger(Baines, 2020; Crouch 2019). Why does increasing the length of telomeres in cells have such a positive impact on longevity?

Research shows that those with shorter telomeres have a poorer survival or shorter lifespan, due to an increase in mortality from heart and infectious diseases. This is because as part of the normal cellular process that occurs in our bodies, as our cells divide, a small portion or bit of the telomere is lost, and the length of telomeres continues to shorten till it reaches a critical length when cellular senescence and or changes that could lead to could to cancer formation or cell death or apoptosis occurs. Senescence occurs when a cell loses its ability to divide and grow, and apoptosis is programmed cell death (Shammas,2011).

This is one of the reasons why telomere length is sometimes seen as a biological clock that can be used to determine the lifespan of a cell and an organism (Shammas,2011). The good news is that there are many lifestyle changes or factors that can affect the length of a telomere.

Some can make the shortening of telomere length occur faster, others can slow the shortening of the telomere faster. When you are consistently doing those things that will help to lengthen your telomere or slow down the shortening of your telomere length as you get older, you are living a more telomeric lifestyle.

Lack of exercise is one of the lifestyle factors that can significantly shorten your telomere length. Therefore, if you choose to spend most of your time sitting down without exercise, you are choosing a less telomeric lifestyle. Increase in moderate physical activity reduces the shortening of telomeres. Research also shows that telomere length is more in active people than inactive people, irrespective of whether the exercise was vigorous or moderate.

According to the CDC an estimated 110,000 deaths per year could be avoided if US adults 40 years and older increased their moderate-to vigorous exercise by even as little 10 minutes more a day. This means increasing your own baseline exercise or physical activity per day by at least 10 minutes. First things first, how many minutes did you spend exercising or staying physically active every day? Keep in mind that the minimum moderate intensity such as walking, that was recommended by the WHO and the CDC is about 150 minutes per week or at least 30 minutes per day for 5 days in a week.

Challenge yourself to be more physically active every day. Whether it is walking more every day, doing more push-ups, jump ropes, hiking, going to the gym, gardening, or regularly doing  sports that you love, your body needs a good balance of daily physical activity to function well. Research and studies indicate that increasing your physical activity can help you live longer.

Though the answer is yes, most people as they get older end up doing less daily physical activity than they should because they are too tired after work or too stressed out by their day-to-day activities to find the time or motivation to move. This is particularly the case for those between 40 and 65 years of age who are already dealing with enormous challenges from raising their families, getting ahead in  their work or careers, taking care of their parents, or managing their relationships and finding time for themselves.

How many minutes of physical activity do you need every week? Most guidelines recommend about 150 minutes per week of moderate physical activity. What does doing 150 minutes of exercise per week mean? It means you are doing about 30 minutes of exercise per day for at least 5 days a week. If your main exercise is walking, it means you are taking about 3000 steps per day since 1000 steps is equal to about 10 minutes of physical activity. Why is increasing your daily physical activity(PA) such an important part of making yourself healthier and living longer as you get older?

Research shows that exercise can help you boost your mood, help you sleep better, help you keep a healthy weight, improve your immune system, digestive function, and your brain health, in addition to its impact the length of your telomere which can help you to slow down on aging and help you live a longer life.

Research also shows that a sedentary lifestyle is considered a significant risk factor for cardiovascular disease while consistently doing more physical activity could be considered a non-pharmacological intervention for improving cardiovascular fitness in healthy and diseased individuals. Increase daily physical activity improves quality of life, reduces body weight, reduces LDL cholesterol, increases HDL cholesterol, increases insulin sensitivity, and helps to prevent pathologic conditions like obesity, atherosclerosis, diabetes, and decreases blood pressure both at rest and during exercise, thus helping to prevent metabolic syndrome and a hypertensive state (Sorriento, Vaia and Iaccarino, 2021)

You should try and increase your physical activity during the day. The goal here is to give your body enough stimulation during the day so that you aren't full of energy at night. You want to make sure you expend your physical energy long before it is time for  your body to rest and ready itself for sleep.

You should attempt to exercise at least four or five times a week for 45 minutes or more per period. You can include walking or something simple like doing jump ropes and push-ups.  If you prefer, you can include strenuous activities such as running as well.
A combination of moderate exercise followed by short bursts of vigorous exercise appears to have the most impact from physical activity for improving cellular and vascular health.

Why is daily physical activity  a good mini habit for your health? According to AMA a study on physical activity and mortality , found that those who had any combination of medium to high levels of vigorous exercise (running, swimming, and bicycling)(75 to 300 minutes per week) and moderate physical activity  (walking, lower-intensity exercise, and weightlifting)(150 t0 600 minutes per week, could have reduction in mortality of 35 to 42 %(Sara Berg, 2023).

How does physical activity affect your cellular and vascular health? As you already know, consistent physical activity helps to increase the length of your telomeres at the cellular level by helping to decrease the rate of shortening of telomeres that occur with age. At the vascular level , exercise protects the endothelium or cells lining the vessels by reducing reactive oxygen species and reducing inflammation by increasing the synthesis of anti-inflammatory cytokines or chemicals and increases the cellular metabolic state by increasing mitochondrial biogenesis and autophagic influx (Sorriento, Vaia and Iaccarino, 2021). Mitochondria are critical to human health and in organs in which damaged mitochondria accumulate more organ damage or disorders occur(Sorriento, Vaia and Iaccarino, 2021).

You can compare mitochondria to the energy source in your house or the batteries in your computers or smart phones or devices. No matter how expensive your phone is or how well the circuit in your computer is you cannot do much with it, when the battery is not working, or the energy source is unreliable or malfunctioning. When the mitochondria or energy packets in your cells malfunction, a lot can go wrong in your mind, body and spirit.

Interestingly research shows that one easy way to fix potential energy problems in your system is more physical activity. Along with running and walking there are several other physical activities that you can add to your daily life to increase your level of physical activity. You can add jump ropes, pushups, and sporting activities to your daily physical activity.

If you discover that you don't have any time to exercise on a regular basis, you should try to sneak in moments of activity into your schedule. Whenever possible, you should take the stairs instead of the elevator, as little things like that will do wonders for your body.

Concentrate on taking the steps you set up in your simple plan for losing weight. If your plan requires walking 60 minutes a day, do it. Do not make excuses. If you are too busy to spare chunks of 60 minutes at a time, then cut it down to 20 minutes or even 15 minutes at a time.

You also have to become more intentional and decisive as you get older. Research has shown that if you were exercising when you were younger then stopped exercising as you got older, you would increase your risk of having a deadly stroke. On the other hand, if you started exercising between 40 and 60 years, you would reduce your risk of having stroke that can significantly reduce your chances of living longer. This shows that it is really never too late to start exercising or form the habit of consistently increasing the level of your physical activity.

Do not think that it is either you are getting everything right or everything is wrong. If you plan to walk 60 minutes a day but due to circumstances beyond your control you were able to do only 25 minutes, you have not failed. Do the 25 minutes that day, then do 95 minutes the next day to make it up. This still makes a total of 120 minutes in two days. On the third day you can go back to 60 minutes a day. Be flexible.

Make sure you keep track of your progress. Get a guide to aging well journal or workbook to help you keep track of your progress. How many steps do you take every day? How many push-ups do you do every day? You can begin with 10 a day then increase it to 20  a day. If you really become good at it , you can do 50 pushups a day. Remember that the goal is to make the exercise as tolerable as you can for yourself. You can simply stick to 20 push-ups a day, ten in the morning then ten in the evening.

Other ways you can increase your physical activity will include walking a little bit more every day or even doing jump ropes. For jump ropes you can begin with 100  a day , then gradually increase it to about 300 jump ropes every day.

For walking you should also park your car around the corner and walk that extra block or two to get to your destination. As you may know, there are many small things you can add to increase the activity in your life. You can do yard work or gardening. Gardening is one of the ways you can stay physically active while getting the stretches that will stay supple and more flexible as you get older. If you can't  have a garden, get a pot of soil and plant tomatoes or simply get indoor plants that you can take care of.

You can even simply decide to do about 7,500 steps to 10,000 steps  per day or walk 2 to 4 miles every day.  Where will you do the walking? You can do it at home, on a treadmill, in a gym or around your neighborhood. Your overall goal here is to have a healthy and well-balanced life by walking every day. How can you make sure your goals are more realistic?

You can do this by setting daily objectives and the actions you can take to achieve those objectives. If you want to lose 10 pounds in one month, what are the daily actions and objectives that can help you accomplish them? Here are some of the ways you can approach that goal.

You can decide to try to lose weight by increasing your physical activity by making no change to your eating habits and your management of your stress-related and emotional challenges. If you want to lose 10 pounds in one month, it means you want to lose 2.5 pounds per week, leading to 10 pounds in 4 weeks. If you used to walk only 5,000 steps a day, can you lose 2.5 pounds in a week? The answer would be No, because 5,000 steps a day would be equal to 35,000 steps a week. Since 1,000 steps a day would burn off about 50 calories, and 4000 steps would burn off 200 calories per day, 35000 steps would only burn off 1750 calories a week and lead to losing 0.5 or half a pound a week.

Research shows that 3,500 calories of energy equal 1 pound, but we need about 2,000 to 2,500 calories of energy for our usual daily activities. Therefore, you would have to starve or fast all day, in addition to exercising to have the energy deficit of 3,500 calories that will allow you to lose one pound a day. This is potentially dangerous, and it is usually not recommended. A less drastic and more sustainable approach would be to eat about 500 calories less a day or about 3,500 calories per week. The recommendation is to sustainably lose 1 to 2 pounds per week.

Instead of trying to rely entirely on exercise to lose weight it is better to combine consistency in daily physical activity with consistency in healthy eating. For example, walking about  10,000 steps a day would allow you to burn off about 500 calories per day, this will be equal to 70,000 steps per week , and burning off about 3,500 calories per week or losing a pound per week. If walking 10,000 steps per day is combined with eating about 500 calories per day, through the compass vam method or simply cutting down on your food portions and under eating.

If you just simply say you will start walking more every day but have no specific activities or strategies for  walking more, you will end up not meeting that goal, and gradually with time you will become discouraged about improving your health and wellness through walking.  Remember that it is your ability to do the daily grind that leads to improvement and progress.

The good news is that you don't actually have to walk 10,000 steps per day to get the longevity benefits from walking. Research has shown that walking about 8,000 steps a day can help to reduce your chances of getting chronic diseases by 51%. A good approach may be to first begin by consistently walking every day, then gradually increase the number of steps you can take daily. You can decide whether it is better for you to walk early in the morning as we recommend or do it in the afternoon during your break or in the evening after you come back from work.

If you want to do more than walking, you can add pushups and jump ropes to your exercise routine. Maybe you can set the goal of doing 200 jump ropes every day. If you haven't done jump ropes before you can start with 50 a day for the first week, then increase it to 100 per day for the next week.

Remember that you need to set simple goals that you have the means to accomplish. Don't set a goal of improving your physical wellness by going to the gym every day when you know you don't like going to the gym and you won't be able to fit going to the gym regularly into your schedule. This will not be a realistic goal for you.

A more realistic way of meeting your goal of regular physical activity for you might be to begin by finding simple but consistent ways to walk for about 30 minutes every day. If you don't have 30 minutes in one block, break up your exercise into 10 or 15 minutes each. Remember that 10 minutes of walking is about 1,000 steps. Since on average people have 2 to 2.5 feet per step, it takes about 2,000 steps to cover a mile. The good news is that you can combine the steps from your formal physical activity period with the steps you take during activities like doing your chores, walking from one meeting to another, gardening or during other outdoor activities, to find out the total number of minutes, steps or miles, you have done in a day.

Don't forget that in order to achieve your goals you must have daily objectives and targets that represent mini steps towards accomplishing your goals or projects, that you actually take or do. Don't allow daily distractions to prevent you from meeting your daily physical activity goals. Always strive to live  an intentional life.

Once you have set realistic goals, write down the daily or weekly activities that will help you achieve them. Write them down in your walking logbook or in your health and wellness journal. This is part of the process of forming positive habits. Choose activities that you can do, otherwise you would merely be in the business of proclamations and proposals.

Where you simply proclaim goals without any concrete steps that will help you to accomplish them. To make your goals a reality you have to consistently apply strategy, effort, process and persistence (SEPP) to achieving your goals.

When you strategize for your goals, you give yourself a chance to identify your skills, deficits, and the risks you need to take to meet your goals. You can enhance your skills in achieving targeted goals by setting objectives, as well as standard and optional activities that will help you meet your goals.

If you do not find time for yourself every day  to exercise and stay physically active, you are indirectly finding them to shorten your lifespan by shortening your cells.

What  is your 30-day physical activity challenge? Your goal should be to walk at least 12,000 cumulative steps per day at the end of your 30-day physical activity challenge. On day one, find out the steps you walked. You can measure your steps per day with a pedometer or with a smart watch and get your average for the first 7 days then challenge yourself to meet up your goal by adding to your average in the next 7 days. Challenge yourself to walk at least 120 minutes every day, 55 minutes in the morning or before noon, 25 minutes in the afternoon  and 45 minutes at night and do

300 jump ropes every other day and at least 20 push ups every other day.  Get and start your garden within the next 30 days or buy at least 5 house plants that you will take care of.

## Form the habit of sleeping well every day

The second key to living longer after 50 is sleeping well every day. Good sleep is part of your physical wellness dimension and part of compass physical profile. How many hours you sleep per day should be part of your vital health numbers. Do you know how many hours of sleep you have every day? If you don't know, do your own 72-hour sleep audit or check your health wellness journal.

Did you know that something as simple as making sure that you sleep 7 to 8 hours a day can help you improve your health and wellness and help you live longer as you get older? Unfortunately, as we get older, especially getting to 40 and above, we start to more consistently run into stress triggers and stress generators that make it more difficult for us to sleep well at night.

According to the CDC, 1 out of 3 adults do not get enough sleep or about 7 hours of sleep every night (CDC, 2016). According to the American Academy of Sleep Medicine and the Sleep Research Society, adults aged 18 to 60, need about 7 hours of sleep every night for great health and well-being. Sleeping less than 7 hours every night predisposes one to more chronic conditions like heart disease, diabetes, stroke, mental stress or depression, and obesity. This is consistent with the research that shows that there is an association between chronic poor sleep quality and an increased risk for age-related disease, mental health deterioration, and dying early (Sabot, Lovegrove, and Stapleton, 2023).

Do you know why having poor sleep predisposes one to poor health? Research shows that inadequate sleep is associated with cellular damage through negative effects on telomere length (Sabot, Lovegrove, and Stapleton, 2023).Research also shows that sleep helps restore the body's nervous, immune, muscular, and skeletal systems. This restorative process is crucial for cognitive functions, such as emotional regulation and memory, and overall health and well-being (Sabot, Lovegrove, and Stapleton, 2023). The other thing to remember is that poor sleep includes the number of hours you have slept, how long it takes you to fall sleep and whether you wake feeling rested or not.

One way most people try to deal with insomnia is to take sleeping pills. However, another option is to increase the amount of physical exercise that you participate in during the day. This is one of the keyways to help you get a good sleep at night. The more active your body is during the day, the more likely you are to relax at night and fall asleep faster.

If you doubt this, watch your children. You will find out that they sleep the most when they have been most busy running around and actively playing all day. They get into bed and fall sound asleep.

With regular exercise you'll notice that your quality of sleep is improved and the transition between the cycles and phases of sleep will become smoother and more regular.  By keeping up your physical activity during the day, you may find it easier to deal with the stress and worries of your life.

**Do you understand that there are ways you can easily use your body clock to achieve optimal health?** The more you understand your body clock the more you will know the best time to wake up, work, clean, plan, eat, and go to sleep.  If you work or play late into the night and end up being drained and confused the rest of the day, then you are ignoring your body clock for sleep, and it can affect your health and productivity at work. Get more hours of sleep, so that you can restore your body clock.

Are you a morning person, afternoon person or night person? A friend of mine who was a night person had a hard time adjusting to waking up at 4.a.m., every morning to catch

---

the 5 a.m. bus that would take him to Los Angeles for his morning shift, until he summoned the courage to ask his supervisor for a change to night shift.

Your body clock has the power to shape your energy levels and activities. Eat at the right time. Don't ignore your body's hunger pangs or warning signals. Eat smart. Watch your portion and increase your variety while eating in moderation. This is another way to take advantage of your body clock when making your eating decision. It will also make you sleep better.

Remember that many factors like your environment, actions and thoughts can affect your body clock. Paying attention to these factors can help you make your life healthier. Why? This is because your body depends on an intricate circadian rhythm to function well. It needs adequate sleep, nutrition, and shelter to stay optimal. It also depends on your priorities and how you schedule your activities.

Do you travel a lot as part of your daily activity? How do you handle travel that may affect your body clock? You have to schedule adequate sleep and rest, so that you do not end up getting stressed out and putting in sub-optimal performance. It can affect your outcome and sense of fulfillment. One way to overcome this is to make relentless transformation your priority.

The more you understand the ways your body clock affects your health and energy level, the more you can share the knowledge with your spouse, friends, and family. This is part of the process of increasing your self-mastery and helping yourself live a longer and healthier life!

Apart from inadequate exercise, the other factors that contribute to poor sleep include watching too much TV and using your mobile devices late at night. This is part of the problem with poor time management. Don't stay up late to watch your favorite show. You may enjoy your show, but you will end up not sleeping well at night. This will not be good for your health and well-being, especially if you are over 50 years old.

Will you have the discipline to refuse your favorite TV shows or Netflix movie because too much screen time can lead to unintended consequences? If you stay up late or play late into the night and end up being drained and confused the rest of the day, then you are ignoring your body clock for sleep, and it can affect your health and productivity at work. Get more hours of sleep, so that you can restore your body clock.

Sometimes we are so caught up in our work, entertainment, and daily activities that we put adequate daily sleep on the back burner. The problem is that if do not sleep well every day, our internal balance gets misaligned and the different organ systems in our body begin to function out of step. This will ultimately lead to more stress and less efficient metabolism that will make you gain weight or sabotage your efforts to maintain a healthy weight and a healthier and longer life.

As we get older, we discover that sleep does not come as readily as in the past.  The other problem is that with more responsibilities and more obligations more people sacrifice or postpone adequate sleep for increased daily activity.  The problem is that inadequate sleep will eventually affect your health and productivity.

What is your 30-day sleep challenge? How many hours of sleep do you have every day? Is it 5 hours a day, 6 hours a day or at least 7 hours a day? Record your first 7 days, then the next 7 days, then try to maintain an average of 7 hours a day at the end of your 30-day challenge. What percentage of days do you sleep at least 7 hours? Is it at least up to 80% of days in your 30-day challenge? While 100% is preferred, 80% at least meets the 80:20 rule.

# Form the habit of managing chronic conditions

The third key to living longer as you get older is managing chronic conditions. Are you healthy or do you simply feel healthy without truly knowing if you are healthy or not? The first step towards managing chronic conditions is to find out if you have chronic conditions. Do you know your numbers? When was the last time you checked your blood pressure or went for a physical?

If you are feeling healthy but your blood pressure is 190/100mmHg and you didn't know it, you're a ticking time bomb for a major life altering or possibly life-ending event like a stroke or heart attack. A few years ago, a 53-year-old man, who was in apparent good health  or felt healthy collapsed and died after a failed resuscitation. Before he died, EMT found out that his blood pressure was 260/150 mmHg , and he had had a heart attack while exercising. His wife, who was with him in the gym when he collapsed, said he has always been in relatively good health and was not on any medications.

This example of someone dying while exercising is important because too many people think that simply because they exercise regularly, eat healthy,  sleep well and have no symptoms, then they must be in good health and do not need to do anything else. This is a wrong and potentially deadly assumption.

You need to know your own numbers. You need to have an idea of the potential illnesses you could be dealing with as you get older based on your family history, past medical history and age group. Do you know the commonest cause of illness or death in your age group as you get older? If you want to live longer, it is important that you pay attention to what has happened or is happening to most people your age. This does not mean that what has happened to others will happen to you, but it does not mean it cannot happen to you or to me.

Each person needs to pay attention to the common causes of death and illness for his or her age group. According to the National Council on Aging (NCOA) the leading causes of death among older people in the US are heart disease, cancer, C0VID-19, stroke, chronic lower respiratory diseases, Alzheimer's, and diabetes (NCOA,2023). The interesting thing about this is that 5 years ago or in 2018, it would not have included COVID 19. This shows one of the reasons why everyone has to remain vigilant. Things change, and we have to learn to take notice and make our own adjustments.

According to the WHO, the leading causes of death among older people, worldwide are heart disease, stroke, chronic obstructive pulmonary disease, and lower respiratory infections (WHO, 2020). We need to keep these leading causes of death or illness in mind when making our own  health and wellness decisions and actions. **Caution is**

**not cowardice, and carelessness is not courage-African proverb.**

If you have not yet done a medical or health checkup or physical in years and you have no idea what your blood pressure is or what your weight, blood sugar or cholesterol level is or you haven't done any of your age-related screening tests, how can say with certainty that you are healthy? You can't. You don't know your numbers.

Yet a lot of people simply assume that because they are not on any medications, they don't have any symptoms of illness, and they haven't been to the doctor in years and are feeling well, then they must be healthy. This is not true. If you don't have concrete data and verified medical opinion telling you that your health status is good, just simply trusting your feeling healthy as evidence of your good health can be dangerous for your health. This is especially true as we get older, when the toll of accumulated health problems like occluding or occluded blood vessels could unexpectedly manifest as a heart attack or stroke in a person of apparent good health.

How many times have you heard about someone who was healthy and working out regularly and  was full of life, who suddenly slumped and died? How many times did the news report also state that the person had high blood pressure but didn't know? One way to help yourself minimize the risk of such an experience is to begin your own journey towards a consistent healthy lifestyle.

Don't use your feelings or intuition alone as evidence for your good health. Get a health assessment done. Go and see your doctor and get some labs done to get a data-based health assessment of your health status.

Let's face it! Most of us think we are very healthy. This is a common thought for young adults and those in middle age. Yet we all know that looks can be deceiving. I am sure you have all heard stories of people who were apparently very healthy then suddenly died from a heart attack or after a "brief illness."

I will share with you how you can improve your heart health. Why did I choose to use improving heart health as an example. It is because as we get older, heart disease which is a chronic condition is one the leading cause of death in the world.

You can improve your heart health by reducing your cardiovascular risk factors. Do you know your blood pressure? Do you know how much sodium you eat daily? This is an example of how knowing your numbers can affect different aspects of your health.

It is very important that every  adult who is interested in living a healthy life learns how to assess his or her cardiovascular risk factors and how to modify those that can be modified. Would you not like to know what is your probability or chances of having a heart attack in the next 10 years? Yes, I would because heart disease is among the leading causes of death for middle-aged men and women in most parts of the world, including the United States and Western Europe.

Even in developing countries like Nigeria the trend toward more deaths related to heart disease is becoming more common. Do you have any friends that suddenly died from heart attack? Do you have any friends, relatives, colleagues, or siblings that unexpectedly had heart attacks and survived? This what I typically call a near death experience (NDE)?

Do you want to have your own NDE, before you begin to take the steps that will help you to reduce your cardiovascular risk factors and improve your own heart health?

You can begin this process by finding out the risk you have for diseases or health conditions that are common to your age, sex, or environment. This is a very important part of helping yourself to live a healthier and longer life! High blood pressure, stroke and heart attack and other related heart diseases are common problems that you could experience as you get older. What are going to do about them?

The problem is that most of us still feel that heart attacks are things that happen to others. We do not feel it will happen to us, so we take little or no precautions to modify our risks for such adverse health events. Factors that are used to calculate your cardiovascular risk factor include:
 *Age
*Sex
*Race
 *Family history of heart disease or diabetes
*Lipid profile as stated above.
 *BMI
*Personality type
Age, sex, and race are factors that cannot usually be changed, but you can use them to calculate your cardiovascular risk points and then convert the points to percentage risk for heart attack over a 10-year period.

Do you know your numbers? Do you know your lipid profile? Do you know your cholesterol level? If you don't know your cholesterol and you are 40 and above you are making a big mistake, because some health associations recommend that people should start doing a check of their cholesterol level from 20 years of age. Knowing your lipid profile is important because you can use it in computing your cardiovascular risk. Your lipid profile includes your triglyceride level, total cholesterol, HDL (High Density Lipoprotein) or good cholesterol, and LDL (Low density Lipoprotein) or bad cholesterol. Do you know changes you can make to eating and healthy living habits that will help you reduce your bad cholesterol (LDL) and increase your good cholesterol(HDL)? This is a way of applying the healthy eating compass challenge to a particular aspect of your health.

Here are two things you can do today that will help you reduce your LDL or bad cholesterol. First, you can add chia seeds to your daily meal. The great thing about chia seeds is that you can add them to almost anything you eat. You can add them to your oatmeal, brown rice, salad, or yoghurt. Chia seeds contain a lot of soluble fibers that can help you lower your cholesterol.

The second thing you can do is to cut down on the number of eggs you eat. Though eggs are rich in protein , eggs also have about 180 mg of cholesterol depending on the size of egg. If you must eat egg, eating white, instead of egg  the yolk will help  you cut down on cholesterol.

What are the benefits of cutting down on LDL? According to the CDC, too much LDL can build up in our blood vessels and lead to the buildup of plaque which can increase the risk of heart disease and stroke. This means that high levels of LDL can affect your vascular health. One of the benefits of cutting down LDL is the reduced risk that follows.  Here is an example of the cardiovascular points for a 45- year-old-man Benjamin with a low HDL(<35) and a cholesterol of 220 and a blood pressure of 130/80  mmHg, who is  not diabetic but smokes. Being a 45-year-old male, would give him 6 points, if he was a woman the points would be 5. An HDL of less than 35 would give him 2 points. Total cholesterol of 220 would be equivalent to 2 points. Smoking would give him 4 points, while a blood pressure of 130/80mmHg is equivalent to 3 points.

This calculation means Joseph has (6+2+2+4+3)=17 points and would translate to at least 29.4% risk of cardiovascular disease(CVD) in 10 years .What does this mean?

According to the Framingham Heart Study, moderate risk is a 10-year CVD risk of less than 10%, moderately high risk is 10-20% and high risk is 20%and above. This means that Benjamin has a high risk for cardiovascular disease. For Benjamin the man in this example, his numbers mean that 29 Page 16 out of 100 people with his risk profile will have a heart attack in the next 10 years This is too high a risk as confirmed by the Framingham Heart Study.

The advantage of finding out your risk factor before having a heart attack is that it gives you an opportunity to take action.

What is the benefit of having high HDL? According to the CDC , HDL or high density lipoprotein helps to move cholesterol from the blood to the liver. This means a higher level of HDL would help to reduce the risk of heart disease and stroke.

For Benjamin he can change his risk for a heart disease by quitting smoking, this will take away,4 points from his 17. Making his HDL 50 and his total cholesterol less than 160, would give him points of (-1), and (0). This means his new total CVD points will be (6+(-1)+0+0+3)=8, which will be equivalent to 6.7%,10-year risk of CVD. Essentially this means that by taking action and modifying his risk factors through eating healthier and quitting smoking, Benjamin reduced his risk of having a heart attack by more than half.

He changed his risk of a heart attack from 29 out of 100 people in 10 years to 7 out of 100 people in 10 years, for people with a similar heart risk profile. Wow! I hope you are as excited as I am; with just a few changes to our eating habits and lifestyle changes we can minimize our risk for a life-

threatening event like a heart attack. Do these numbers and percentages look confusing or interesting?
Do not worry, it is not that confusing. You can calculate your own personal risk of having a heart attack by visiting http://hp2010.nhlbihin.net/atpiii/calculator.asp

I am certainly looking forward to sharing simpler, fast, and easy ways you can develop a blueprint that will help you transform your overall health and wellness. Healthy eating is one factor that can help you improve your heart health. Remember to eat more fruits and vegetables like apples, cucumbers and colorful vegetables that can help you improve your heart health. At the end of this training, you have to decide to consistently apply the 80:20 rule to your heart health. Decide to apply the 80:20 rule to your exercise regimen.

This means you have to decide and follow through on doing consistent physical activity. Don't try to do everything. Find 1 out of 5 and do it 80% of the time. Walking is strongly recommended. The other is healthy eating. Don't try to eat all veggies and fruits, find about 3 of 15 that you eat 80 % of the time. Make sure you actually eat something  you actually like. An example would be making sure you eat broccoli, cucumbers, apples, oranges, and grapes. If you can't them eat directly, make them into smoothies and drink them. Finally make sure you also apply the 80:20 rule to maintaining your own positive and supportive relationships and improving your self-care

What is your 30-day managing chronic conditions challenge? First write down the chronic conditions that you know of in the first 7 days. If you don't of any, start by checking your blood pressure and weighing yourself.  The second step is to go to your doctor and find out if you have any chronic conditions that you may unknowingly have. At the end of the 30-day challenge, you will know how many of the steps recommended in this chapter have been consistently doing

## Eat healthy by making healthy food choices and eating in moderation

**The fourth key to living longer after 50 is to eat healthy by making healthy food choices and eating in moderation.** While there are many ways to make healthy food choices or eat healthy, I will share with you how to use the compass VAM method and to eat healthy.

Why would making healthy food choices and eating in moderation help you to live longer? According to the Global Burden of Disease study, 1 in 5 deaths in the world can be prevented by eating healthy or improving the quality of diet. One way to simply do this is to eat more plant-based food and cut down on processed food.

According to CDC sugar-sweetened beverages (SSBs) or sugary drinks like sodas are leading sources of added sugars in the American diet. Drinking soda is associated with weight gain/obesity, type 2 diabetes, gout, tooth decay, heart disease, kidney diseases, and liver disease (CDC, 2017). If you want to live longer one of the healthy food choices you can make is to cut down on drinking sugary drinks or sugar-sweetened beverages like soda, fruit juice, and fruit punch. **Drink water or unsweetened tea instead of soda.**

Do not go along with food choices that will not be good for your health just because your friends, members of your family, co-workers or people from your culture may challenge you or make fun of you. Your culture is supposed to help you, not to kill you. You can do this by finding a way to eat right within your culture or while hanging out with your friends and co-workers.

**The first thing to remember is that eating healthy will you help maintain a healthy weight, which can help you to reduce the effect of being overweight or obese on your lifespan.** Research shows that having excessive weight can lead to increase in insulin resistance, inflammation, and metabolic and hormonal changes that can lead to neurodegeneration, atherosclerosis and a tendency to produce tumors.

Research also shows that increasing body mass index (BMI) increases the risk of developing type 2 diabetes, cancer and cardiovascular disease. In addition to being associated with the above listed changes, having excessive fat which is both a function of how you eat and how consistently you exercise can increase the risk of having coronary disease, high blood pressure, nonalcoholic liver disease, stroke , type 2 diabetes and aging at a faster rate.

Have you done your 72- hour food audit to get an idea of the food choices you typically make? What did you eat last night? Do you eat a lot of processed food? If you haven't done your 72 – hour food audit, do it or go back to your  health and wellness journal to find out your eating pattern and food choices. This will help you decide the changes you need to make to help you eat healthy and make the food choices that will help you live a healthier and longer life.

Do you remember exactly what you were doing at this time yesterday? Did someone make you eat too much, or did you resist and eat right? Do you weigh yourself every week? If you weigh yourself every week, it will help you keep your weight healthy by keeping better track of your weight or changes to your weight. This way you can catch negative trends early and begin to make changes early.

Get a weight-loss journal or notebook. Unless you have a way to regularly evaluate your progress throughout your health and wellness  loss journey, you will find sustainable success more difficult to maintain. How can you tell if you are meeting your daily mini goals if you don't evaluate yourself? Evaluating yourself regularly and taking daily positive action will help you form the right healthy habits.

The more you know about how unhealthy food choices can affect your weight, cellular and vascular health, the more you will be interested in making sustainable lifestyle changes. Do you regularly eat your variety vegetables and fruits? If you truly want to maintain a healthy weight you have to eat more plant-based food like fruits, vegetables and nuts. Can you name the top 5 fruits and vegetables that you like? Do you eat them every week?

Do you eat cucumbers, cabbages, green leaf, tomatoes, broccoli, oranges, mangoes, apples, pineapples, grapes, and blueberries? If these do not work for you,  make your own list. Make changes for the ones you don't like. Some people prefer carrots to mangoes. Make your own list and regularly eat them or regularly make fruit and vegetable smoothies from them.  You can try the blueberry and cucumber smoothie made with grapes and bananas. It is delicious and smooth!

Do you know that the kind of self-talk you give yourself can affect your weight? This is part of the process of autosuggestion with which you can direct your subconscious mind. If you tell yourself that you can't lose weight, then you will find a way to gain weight even  after you have started losing weight or started making the right adjustments.

Remember that it is easier to watch your portion and reduce 100 calories food intake, than it is to exercise and burn off the 100 calories that you have eaten. Do you still exercise regularly or have discovered that "you don't have time"? Are you becoming better at managing stress that could arise out of your interactions, conversations, and relationships with yourself and others?

To lose weight and keep it off you have to be able to measure and demonstrate to yourself that what you are doing is working. Weigh yourself at least once a week. Measure your waist circumference. Take time to fill in your compass healthy living logbook or journal every week.

This will give you an idea of some factors contributing to your weight gain or stubborn weight loss. Maybe you are spending too much time watching TV or on social media. According to Cleland, Schmidt, Dwyer, &Venn, the (2008) time spent in behaviors that involve a lot of sitting with little activity, like watching or viewing TV was thought to be one of the factors responsible for increasing number of people that are either overweight or obese in different parts of the world. The study also found that in both men and women the average time spent watching television increased with the increasing frequency of consuming food and drinks while watching television. Soft drink consumption during television viewing was associated with a greater increase in abdominal obesity in both men and women.

**After you have determined or discovered the easy activities that will consistently help you to lose weight, take realistic action to transform yourself and get the results you want for yourself.** Your goals should be achievable in the context of the circumstances of your life and how far you want to go in terms of living a healthier and longer life.

One way to check your progress in your weight loss journey is to take regular measurements. You can do this by weighing yourself every week, measuring your waist circumference every month, and calculating your BMI every three months. You can also use less formal ways like dress size, change in belt hole, pant size, loose ring, or changes in shoe fitting to evaluate your weight loss journey.

Weigh yourself before you start then weigh yourself after every week. You can use a simple scale to weigh yourself. Measuring your weight regularly is one of the easiest checks on how your individualized health plan is working. It is easier to do than calculating your BMI or measuring your waist circumference. Just climb on a scale and read your weight.

If on the other hand you discover that you have gained back some of the weight you have lost, then do a quick 72 –hour food audit to see the eating patterns that are making you gain weight. Short-term weight gains usually are as a result of increasing calorie intake or eating more food, rather than simply from reducing physical activity.

**Remember that a lapse is not a relapse. A mistake is not a failure. Don't be too harsh on yourself !** If you find yourself not sticking to the eating patterns that can help you eat more fruits and vegetables, think about trying out new changes that you have not tried in the past. Talk to your support group and share your ideas on eating time and food variety. Do you know how many times Thomas Edison did not succeed or failed, before he finally succeeded? 999 times!!!

Try again if you do not succeed the first time. If you are living by yourself and are no longer in touch with your family or old friends, create a new support group or join one online. Are you becoming better at managing stress that could arise out of your interactions, conversations, and relationships with yourself and others?

Get a weight-loss journal or notebook. Unless you have a way to regularly evaluate your progress throughout your health and wellness loss journey, you will find sustainable success more difficult to maintain. How can you tell if you are meeting your daily mini goals if you don't evaluate yourself? Evaluating yourself regularly and taking daily positive action will help you form the right healthy eating habits.

**Do not forget to talk to your doctor or health care provider about your medications. Make sure you are not taking any medications or have any underlying disorders that may make you gain weight.** This is particularly important if through a chart of your weekly weight measurement you discover that you have gained weight.

Check your list of activities you consider realistic for you to accomplish your weight loss in a day based on your knowledge, experience, personality, available resources, and your stress management skills. Once you have a concrete list in front of you, it's a lot easier to check on yourself regularly and know what lifestyle changes you will need to make.

One of the lifestyle changes that you can make as you get older is to eat healthy by making healthy food choices and eating in moderation. At the Compass Wellness Institute, the recommendation is to use the compass VAM method, which is a combination of the compass intermittent fasting healthy eating plan and eating in moderation through VAM. If you want to use the compass intermittent healthy eating plan , please make sure you talk to your doctor or provider first.

Please don't do intermittent fasting without first talking to your doctor or provider. Don't do intermittent fasting if you are trying to conceive, pregnant or nursing. Intermittent fasting is broadly defined as any diet or eating plan that includes regular periods of not eating or fasting.

While there are many ways to do intermittent fasting, what we use and encourage others to use is the 16:8 type of intermittent fasting. In this type you fast for 16 hours then you eat in 8 hours. Though it is hard to eat too much in 8 hours, it is still a possibility, especially risk  if you do not apply the compass VAM method to the eating  part of after you have fasted for 16 hours. When you are following the 16:8 intermittent fasting type, you will fast for 16 hours a day, and have the remaining 8 hours to eat. With intermittent fasting you can easily cut down your caloric intake without counting calories. Intermittent fasting has also been found to be one of the healthy, safe and easy ways to lose 1-2 lbs. per week.

The 5:2 intermittent fasting type involves eating regularly for 5 days, with fasting or eating very little for 2 days.  The intermittent fasting type that we use in the compass healthy intermittent eating plan is the 16;8 type or approach.

Research shows that intermittent fasting works by extending the time the body has burned through the calories consumed in your last meal and begins to burn fat in lieu of consumed calories (John Hopkins, 2022).

You have to remember that the period of fasting could lead to even more hunger pangs, tiredness, loss of concentration, and weakness. The good news is that during the fasting period, you can drink water, black coffee, and unsweetened tea. Personally, I start my day with black coffee, it helps to keep me sharp and alert as I go through my day.

You will require some discipline to make sure that you manage the hunger pangs during the fasting period well. Don't drink soda or eat many hot dogs as an immediate way of dealing with your hunger pangs. This could only lead to breaking the fast and failing to get the full benefits of intermittent fasting.

One of the biggest mistakes people make is that after the fasting phase of intermittent fasting, they eat too much during the eating phase. They fail to watch the portion of the food they eat, the type of food they eat and the servings of fruits and vegetables that they eat. This is a challenge that you have to decide to overcome in the heathy eating step of the compass challenge.

You must decide that eating healthy is an important part of your journey towards living a healthier and longer life. Remember that research has shown that eating healthy is one of the ways you can potentially reduce the shortening of the length of telomeres in your cells, leading to delayed onset of age-related diseases and increased longevity or lifespan (Shamas,2011).You can make changes to your eating habits through the compass vam method.

Make sure you don't eat too much during the eating phase of intermittent fasting. If you eat too much during that phase, it will defeat the purpose of your fasting phase, because you would simply have more energy intake and more weight gain. Adjustments are changes you make to your eating pattern and your meals so that you can continue to lose weight or maintain a healthy weight and live a healthier and longer life.

**VAM stands for variety, adjustments, and moderation**. The order in which you make the modifications is entirely up to you. A suggested first strategy would be for you to start by reducing the food portion of your daily meals. **The first step towards implementing your compass "VAM" method for relentless weight loss is to cut down the servings or portions of your regular meal by half.** This will reduce your energy intake by about half or a third. You fill the gap with vegetables and fruits. If you feel pangs of hunger, snack with nuts, drink plenty of water or eat some fruits.

Why is the reduction in portions so important? According to surveys by doctors and nutritionists the average American male takes about 3,000 calories per day and the American female about 2,400 calories per day (Reuters Health, 2015). According to Dr. Wang an energy intake and expenditure expert, consistent loss, or reduction in energy intake of 100 calories would lead to 10 pounds loss in weight (Reuters Health, 2015). **This means that without knowing the exact quantity of calories you eat, you**

**can continue to reduce your meal, snack, or social eating portions until you notice your first loss of 10 pounds and use it for a marker or foundation for all your future weight-loss strategies.**

The more you reduce your servings, the more weight you would lose because the fewer calories you will take in, the less excess calories you will have to store as fat. However, reduced servings may mean more hunger pangs. This is a serious potential problem that could make you drink a lot of soda or eat many hot dogs as an immediate way of dealing with your hunger pangs. Unless you make adjustments, this could simply lead you to more energy intake and more weight gain.

**The next step in the compass vam method is to make adjustments.** Adjustments are changes you make to your eating pattern and your meals so that you can continue to eat healthy and maintain a healthy weight. If you truly want to succeed in living a healthy and longer life, you must make the adjustments that fit into your world view, self and spiritual compass profiles.

What are the patterns you commonly encounter in your daily life? Write down the patterns that are most prominent in your life in the past 72 hours or 7days. You can write this down in your "Guide to Aging Well" journal or Wellness journal. Identify and write down the following with regards to you:

*Eating pattern
*Working pattern
*Communication pattern
*Decision making pattern
*Relationship pattern
* Stress pattern
*Conflict pattern
*Activity pattern
*And Meditation pattern.

Why are patterns important? Through them you will get a better idea of the habits that are driving your daily action and Lifestyle. Through the answers to the following questions, you find your own eating pattern:

What did you have for breakfast or lunch 2 days ago? Was it healthy? Was it more plant-based or more processed food?

What about lunch? Was it more processed food? What type of food do you like? What about fruits and vegetables?

What did you eat for supper? When did you eat your number? Did you drink water or soda with your meal?

Did you snack on fruits, cookies, chips, or candy? Do you eat snacks just before you go to bed?

How would you cope with any challenges or negativity that your own daily patterns may have revealed? Do you cope with your daily challenges by drinking alcohol, smoking eating more food or watching porn? Can you give up alcohol and smoking by making  the adjustments that help you  live a healthier and longer life?

Can you make adjustments to how many cans of soda  you drink every day? Drinking more soda is the wrong **adjustment** for hunger pangs from portion reduction. The right **adjustment** would be to eat more fruits, vegetables, and fibers as fillers. Fibers are especially good for your system because they help to increase bowel movement. This has the added effect of making your digestive system more efficient.

**Sometimes the adjustment you can make will be affected by your culture. For different cultures and settings, different modifications to familiar eating habits can be made. In the United States this would entail cutting down on fast foods, soda, and other processed foods.**

According to the CDC sugar-sweetened beverages (SSBs) or sugary drinks like sodas are leading sources of added sugars in the American diet. Drinking soda is associated with weight gain/obesity, type 2 diabetes, gout, tooth decay, heart disease, kidney diseases, and liver disease (CDC, 2017). If you want to live longer of the healthy food choices you can make to drinking sugary drinks or sugar-sweetened beverages like soda, fruit-juice, and fruit punch. **Drink water or unsweetened tea instead of soda.**

Do not go along with food choices that will not be good for your health just because people from your culture may challenge you or make fun of you. Your culture is supposed to help you, not to kill you. You can do this by finding a way to eat right within your culture. If you cannot completely eliminate fast food cut it down to once a month.

**Another adjustment could be to stop eating processed food like bread.** Did you know that bread can be a source of sodium and too much energy intake? Did you know that on average a slide of bread contains 150 mg of sodium and 110 calories per serving? This would mean that for bread with one slice per serving, 10 slices would be 1100calories. This would be more than half of the average 2000 calories per day recommended for most people.

Are you struggling to control your weight?

Do you know why you have gained weight though you're exercising more? If you are eating in moderation by cutting down your portions, eating fruits and vegetables and doing regular exercise but have not lost weight, you wonder why.

The first reason may be because you have not cut down on the daily amount of sugar you eat every day. Though the recommended daily sugar intake for men is about 36 g or 9 teaspoons and 25 g or 6 teaspoons for women, Americans eat about 3 times this value everyday (AHA). This is because most people end up eating varieties of candy and drinking soda every day.

Did you know that in the past 30 years more and more sugar has been added the American diet (AHA)? The more sugar you eat the more calories you shall eat that will make you continue to gain weight despite the reduction in portion size and increase in exercise. Make sure before you eat that you check the Nutrition Facts in every food that you eat. Make sure you always check for added sugar in what you eat.

The second reason may be related to your snacking habits. Did you know that one small pack of unsalted pea nuts contained 220 calories per serving but 6 servings per pack? How does this information which you read from the nutrition facts on the pack help you? It can help you determine calories per pack, sodium per pack and sugar per pack.

Be careful with snacks!!! Did you know that when you finish a pack of pea nuts rich in dietary fiber, with little or zero sodium and cholesterol, you are also eating more than 1000 calories. When you combine it with 1100 calories from 10 slices of bread, it means that from bread and peanuts alone, give you have more than 2000 calories already eaten (1100+1320=2420) calories. This shows that though you had reduced your calories per meal through reducing your portion per meal, because you had not paid careful attention to size or frequency of your snacks, you were still eating a lot of calories per day through snacks.

**Managing your weight has to be part of your health and wellness journey. If you want to lose weight and keep it off, you have to know your daily sources of extra calories. Do you know how many calories you have in your morning cereal or pack of pea nuts?** When you regularly read the nutritional facts in the food you eat, you can find out calories per serving. When you know the calories per serving you can more realistically adjust your portion size to cut down on your daily calories intake without counting calories.

If you are eating a lot of nuts, check your nutritional facts as soon as possible. When I checked mine, I discovered that I was eating more calories through my snacks than I expected. I cut my snack portions by more than half. This helped me reduce my extra calories by more than half. This adjustment helped me to start losing weight more consistently and keeping it off. You can do the same or something similar, after a full examination of your own snacking habits. You don't have to cut your calories by half, you can begin with a third, then reduce your snacks by more as you make more adjustments.

**You do not have to do a full detailed calories count to know your average energy intake. You can get a good idea of your calories intake by doing your own 72-hour food audit. This will help you identify the highest and most frequent source of calories in your daily meals.**

**All you have to do is to remember that you have to reduce all sources of your daily intake of calories from your meals to your snacks. Do this to a level that allows you to feel full, eat healthy and still lose weight. Remember  that it is calories in, calories out!**

Apart from the adjustments I have mentioned so far, another easy one you can quickly do is to start drinking a glass of water before each meal. This will make feel full, without eating as much as before. After a while, you will be able to consistently cut down on your daily portions of food or snacks.

Another healthy food choice you make is to drink at least one glass of water before you eat. Research has shown that drinking water before a meal will help to expand your stomach. This approach will make you feel completely full when you are only 80% full. This is important because eating only up to 80 % full was one of the common practices of people of Okinawa in Japan, who have the highest number of centenarians in the world (Boyle & Long, 2010).

Okinawa is one of the so-called blue zones in the world where a lot of people live up to 100 years or more. If you want to lose weight or manage your weight better without making it seem like a tedious task, then drink at least two glasses of water per meal and increase the bulk in your meals through fruits and vegetables. **This will help you reduce your total calorie intake per meal without torture diets or counting calories.**

First, based on your 72 – hour health and wellness audit, how many servings of fruits and vegetables do you eat in a week? Is it 15 servings per week, based on 3 servings per day? To increase your intake of fruits and vegetables, start by eating every meal with salads consisting of cabbage, tomatoes, carrots, broccoli, bananas, and spinach. Eating a colorful variety of vegetables and fruits per meal with quinoas or reduced portions of brown rice or complex carbs like oatmeal or kinos will make your meal significantly more healthy and bulkier but less energy dense. It will help you to lose significant pounds and keep them off. **Remember calories in calories out. However, it is better when those calories contain fibers too.**

You need to be careful when you start cutting down on calories by reducing the intake of carbohydrates like white bread, white rice, or pasta. This will make you lose weight quickly because it is usually stored in the body as glycogen which contains water. You need to be careful because the brain gets most of its energy from glucose and if it does not get enough you begin to feel tired, weak, unable to sleep and unable to focus.

This is one of the reasons why it is important to remember that when it comes to healthy living everything is interrelated. Go back to your 72-hour health and wellness audit to check how other factors affect what you eat. How many hours of sleep do you have per day? If you don't sleep well , you will be tired during the day and will not find your days as enjoyable as you would like them to be.

How much stress do you have to deal with every day? How positive are your interactions with others? How consistently do you strive to be intentional in everything you do? Do you smoke? What habits do you use to strive to become a better version of yourself? Do you drink alcohol? Do you do drugs?

How much fiber do you eat daily? Unless you switch to fiber-rich carbohydrate sources like baked sweet potato, whole grain bread, barley, oatmeal, and brown rice, you may end up quitting after a few weeks. Should you make your food choices based on their glycemic index or fiber content?

Glycemic index is a measure of the blood glucose -raising potential of the carbohydrate content of a food compared to a refence food (typically pure glucose). GI 70 or more is high, and 56 to 69 is moderate, while 55 and less is low. The interesting thing about deciding whether you are going to eat low glycemic index (GI)foods or high fiber foods is that most foods that are high fiber are also low GI foods. It's almost like looking at different ways of getting the same result, which is eating healthy.

Generally speaking, the more processed food you eat, the higher the GI of the food you are eating. While it is good to know about different ways, what we eat can impact our health, sometimes when you find a way to eat healthy that verifiably works for you without the knowledge of all other terms and ways of classifying healthy food, what may matter more is your consistency in eating right. Fast when you can or when it is safe for you do so and make more of your food more plant-based, while watching portions and snacks

Some examples of low GI foods include apples, blueberries, prunes, cranberries, pinto beans, green beans, lentils, non-vegetables like broccoli, spinach, tomatoes, cabbage, asparagus, tomatoes, cabbage, and avocado. Other low GI foods include almonds, peanuts, skinless chicken, turkey, almond milk, skim milk, and fish. Interestingly, I have been eating peanuts, broccoli, turkey, apples, and bananas, without checking either glycemic index or glycemic load. Does that mean that I am not making healthy food choices? No. Does everyone need to know the GI and GI of every food they eat before they can eat healthy? No. Having an idea is good but not necessary as long as you focus on eating plant-based food and cutting down on proceeds food and red meat.

**To make sustainable adjustments and modifications to your meals, concentrate on variety and moderation.** Include chicken, fish, beans, cottage cheese, chia seeds or low-fat yogurt in your meals. You can make low fat yogurt and chia seeds for your breakfast. Have eggs, nuts, and red meat occasionally. By occasionally, I mean about 2 times a week. Eat fish at least once a week. How many times do you eat fish every week?

You can further reduce your fat intake by eating skinless chicken or turkey. Turkey and chicken have their fat on their skin, but red meat has most of its fat contained within the meat. Grilling is better than frying.

Always aim to use unsaturated oils like corn, and olive oils for cooking. Do you prefer frying to grilling? Why is this even important to consider? Grilling does not add additional fat or calories to your food. Do you prefer frying to grilling? Why is this even important to consider? It is important because of the relationship between Advanced glycation end products(AGEs) our health, and how food is prepared. According to the NIH, most modern food and related meals are made by heating food , leading to  dietary AGEs that contribute to oxidant cellular damage and chronic inflammation that contribute to heart and vascular disease and metabolic disorders like diabetes. AGEs bind to cell surfaces and body proteins affecting cellular and organ function.

Foods rich in protein and fat contain more AGEs than those rich in carbohydrates such as fruits, vegetables, and whole grains. Foods fried tend to have more AGEs than food that is grilled. Part of the reason is that fried food tends to have more fat added as part of the process of preparing the food through frying.

You can also gradually reduce the fat content in your milk products. You can do this by changing the variety of milk that you drink from whole milk to 2% fat: then to 1% fat. I am wary of fat free milk because it is still important to get fat in your body which can be used through cellular metabolism to produce cell membranes and hormones. Choose lower-fat cheese and yogurt. When you buy yogurt, also check that it does not contain sugar. The good thing about reducing to 1% fat milk is that it remains tasty. Fat has 9 calories of energy per gram compared to carbohydrates and proteins that have about 4 per gram.

**Remember that variety is the spice of life. It is the "V" in the compass vam method.** Do not eat the same meal day in day out. Why? It gets boring after a while, and you will soon find yourself looking less excited about eating healthily. You have to like and enjoy what you eat. **Healthy eating is not punishment!**

**To sustainably manage your holistic wellness, you have to aim for a healthy variety of food that contains adequate but moderate portions of fat, proteins, carbohydrates and vitamins.** Eat enough food to fill full when you eat. If you don't feel full after a meal you will find yourself eating too many sugary snacks in between meals to make you feel full. One trick is to drink a glass of water before every meal, it will help you to feel more full with every meal.

If you feel full after a meal you may find yourself with so much food in between meals that you may begin to gain back weight that you may have lost. If you feel hungry between meals, snack small portions of almonds, cashew nuts or peanuts. Almonds will make you feel less hungry and still boost your metabolism, though they take getting used. Have you tried almonds before?

The challenge is that sometimes even when you know what is right to do or eat, doing it consistently can be a problem. This is part of reason why I always suggest that you have at least 3 go to nuts that you can rely on, to use as snacks in -between meals. My own go-to nuts are peanuts, almonds, and cashew nuts all unsalted. What are yours?

**The third part of VAM is variety. Make variety part of your daily eating habit.** Do not eat a particular food too much just because you like it. If usually eat  a lot of white bread and soda just because you enjoyed them, cut down your portions then consider stopping them altogether. This is because bread and soda contain significant calories and sodium.

Strictly speaking, you have to watch how much soda or beer you drink. Beer has a lot of empty calories with little ingredients. Drinking too much beer may increase your belly fat without giving you adequate amounts of important vitamins like vitamin B 6.

Another way to balance your meal would be to halve or significantly cut down on  your intake of all pure or added fats as previously outlined. If you are not sure, check the types of food that you have been eating based on your last 72-hour health and wellness or food audit.

**If you plan your meals and snacks ahead of time you will have to make them the variety that will help you to stay heathy and counter the effects of oxidants and chronic inflammation on your body.** Take time to plan at least one lunch and dinner every week without meat or cheese and eat more fruit.

Create your meals around whole grains, vegetables, and beans to increase fiber and reduce fat. If you want to have something to chew on, get some fish or tofu. You can make every Friday your fish meal day to begin with then gradually add more and more fish to your meals.

**Have at least five servings of fruit and vegetables every day.** Choose fruit that is in season. Take an apple per meal. The red delicious apples contain pectin, a fiber that helps to promote healthy cholesterol levels and contain more amounts of antioxidants than many other types of apples.

Do you eat cucumbers every day? Make them part of your daily meal. According to the USDA  cucumbers on average contain about 2.8mg sodium and about 193mg of potassium, Vitamin K, Lutein and Zeaxanthin , Ig of fiber and cucurbitacins. Research has shown that cucurbitacin's help to fight liver, breast, lung, and prostate cancer by helping to stop cancer cells from multiplying or growing. On the other hand, the  high potassium and very low sodium content of cucumber helps it to reduce blood pressure. Potassium generally helps to lower blood pressure because of its effect on blood vessels and how it counteracts the effect of sodium.

These are just a few examples of how fruits and vegetables, and healthy eating in general can help you live a heathier and longer life. However, keep in mind that all the depth of knowledge and insight into eating food that will help you maintain a healthy weight and improve your health will only work if you take consistent positive daily action! Use the tips and strategies on the compass vam method shared with you in this chapter to develop your own healthy eating blueprint. Make sure you keep to the healthy-eating blue print you have developed at least 80 percent of the time! This way you can use the 80:20 rule as your guard rails in your wellness and longevity journey.

Here are a few more tips on what you can do to help you live a healthier and longer life.

*Cut down your food portions by at least one-third.

---

# 8 Keys To Longevity  After  50

*Drink low-fat milk or eat low fat yoghurt.

*Eat at one least one cucumber per day.

*Eat at least five servings of fruits and vegetables daily.

*Eat your food in one location without TV or without your smart phone.

*Eat at least one quarter of a watermelon every day

*Eat fish and skinless poultry like chicken or turkey at least once a week.

*Eat only 80% of your meal

*Do you keep to the healthy-eating blue print you have developed , at least 80percent of the time?

*Keep eating right even after a lapse.

What is your 30-day challenge goal for eating healthy and losing weight or maintaining a healthy weight? How many times did you eat 80 percent of your meal? Did you drink water before every meal? Assess your first week and see if you are at least 80 percent closer to the mark you set for yourself, then become more consistent towards the end of your 30-day challenge.

# Form the habit of effectively managing stress every day

Managing stress effectively every day is the fifth key to longevity. Remember that everything is interrelated and without vigilance you can easily get distracted, disrupted, or discouraged by stress. Any one of your daily interactions can become a stressor because it can alter the balance or homeostasis within your body system. After all, stress can be defined as a threat to homeostasis or inner balance caused by a variety of stressors, such as environmental, psychological, or physiological factors (Chung, 2005)

How can poorly managed stress affect your health and longevity? Stress can exert various actions on the body ranging from alterations in homeostasis to life-threatening effects and death. Stress  can either be a triggering or aggravating factor for many diseases and pathological conditions (Yaribeygi et al, 2017).

Research shows that stress increases the risk of diabetes mellitus, can lead to build up of plaque in arteries(atherosclerosis), especially if combined with unhealthy eating and a sedentary lifestyle, and can lead to anxiety, depression, and severe broncho-constriction in asthmatics (Salleh, 2008). How does stress affect your cellular and vascular health or your ability to live a healthier and longer life?

Depending on the severity and duration of stress, the cells in our bodies can either re-establish homeostasis or adapt to an altered state or cell response that leads to adaptation, autophagy, or cell death. Stress can affect cellular health by leading to damage to proteins, organelles like mitochondria or the powerhouse of cells, DNA, RNA, or lipids. The accumulation of damaged macromolecular from persistent stress or repeated acute stress in our cells can lead to degenerative diseases, cardiovascular diseases, malignancies, and

contribute to the process of aging (Poljšak and Milisav, 2012 ; Chung, 2005 ).
One of the ways stresses can affect your vascular health is due to the enhanced activation of your sympathetic nervous system, which can lead to inflammation of your vessels, leading to increase in platelet adhesion and aggregation, atherosclerosis, thrombosis, and activation of macrophages (Chung, 2005).

The other way stress affects cellular and vascular health is that stress through the flight or fight response, through the effect on the brain and glands in the body(HPA axis) induces the secretion of glucocorticoids and adrenaline (stress hormones) that generation of reactive oxygen species(ROS) that cause increased mitochondrial activity and increased damaging and shortening of. Telomeres. Damaged and shortened telomeres are associated with chronic inflammation and age-related degenerative diseases (Lin and Epel, 2022).

Why should you care about the effect of stress on the length of telomeres? Research found that those 60 years and above with shorter telomere length had earlier all-cause mortality from infectious disease and heart disease (Lin and Epel, 2022).When you are thinking of how stress affects your cellular and vascular health and your ability to live a long and healthy life, remember that stress can shorten your telomeres and through stress hormones can predispose you to cellular changes, and chronic inflammation that lead to disease and possibly early death. Please don't just simply dismiss stress or your daily stressors as nothing.

Research also shows that emotional stress contributes significantly to cancer, cardiovascular disease, accidental injuries, respiratory disorders, liver cirrhosis, and suicide, which are among the leading causes of death in the United States (Salleh,2008). Are you mentally focused enough to maintain your peace of mind and protect your health every day?

Don't assume that because you do not have high blood pressure, diabetes, or any other leading cause of death, then you are fine, and you don't have to do anything. You must remain vigilant. Research shows that that even in individuals with normal blood pressure a tendency to anger can increase the risk to CAD(acute myocardial infarction(MI)/fatal CAD, silent MI, or cardiac catheterization procedures) and hard events(acute MI/fatal CAD) compared to those a lower tendency to anger (Chung,2005). The good news is that the more you learn about how to stay calm under pressure, and how to manage stress better, the more you can keep anger and the related consequences out of your system.

How stress will affect you depends on whether you have the resources to cope with the problem generating the stress, your genetic vulnerability, coping style, personality, and social support. The first step towards managing stress more effectively in your daily life as you get older is to do your own 72-hour stress audit so that you can find the most common stressors you have to deal with. You can also find out the most common causes of stress in your life by reviewing your health and wellness journal or your guide to aging well workbook.

How do you manage daily stress that can arise from disruptive interactions? How do you manage stress that arises from minor incidents or conversations? Do you lash out in anger? How do you manage conversational stress? How do you manage interactional or emotional stress? If you want to remain on track in your health and wellness journey throughout your daily interactions with others, you must be able to consistently deal with daily stress, no matter what.

Despite all these factors that affect how stress will affect you, it is ultimately your way of reacting to stress that will determine your susceptibility to illness and your overall health and wellness (Salleh,2008). **This means you must learn to stay calm under pressure and stay fully immersed in the moment.** One way is to recognize challenges associated with daily conversations or interactions that could lead to disruptive tangents. It is wise sometimes to think about both a positive or negative response before you ask a question or begin a conversation.

While you might have had an idea about some of the common causes of stress in your life during your 72-hour health and wellness audit, doing a more specific 72-hour stress audit will give you a better idea of the factors that lead to stress in your life. It could be your thoughts, your conversations, your ambitions or your situation and circumstance. Are you dealing with a toxic work environment, home environment or social environment?

How do you deal with daily hassles such as arguments at work, at  home, or at events, annoying drivers, marital problems, financial difficulties, and challenges at work which could be sources of repeated acute stress or sources of chronic stress?

You can use mind over matter to manage stress. After all, according to Marcus Aurelius, "A real man doesn't give way to anger and discontent, and such a person has strength, courage, and endurance-unlike the angry and complaining. The nearer a man can come to a calm mind, the closer he is to strength." Don't let the perfect become the enemy of the possible while you are striving to be the best version of yourself in all aspects of your life.

If you closely analyze  the common sources of stress in your life you will discover that 20% of the causes or 1 out of 5 of the common causes of stress will be responsible for 80 % of the stress that you will deal with every day. How can which ones with certainty? Check the entries you have made in compass stress journal.

How can you become better at managing common causes of stress in your daily life and stay calm under pressure? Mastery over daily moments  is part of the skills you need to learn in order to reduce and manage stress and anxiety in your daily life. You must remember that at every point in time you are interacting with another person, and that person may be dealing with other factors that could be interacting with them.

This could be affecting their own personal situation and the circumstances in which they find themselves. It is like a driver who was thinking of what to do after being unexpectedly fired at the office, then fails to stop at the stop sign, then crashes into another car that had the right of way. Do you think that driver was thinking of his driving at the moment of the crash or was thinking of the fact that he had just been fired at the moment of the crash?

This is why even in the smallest interactions with others, other things can go wrong in the blink of an eye, even when it is least expected. If this happens to you, don't take it personally. Remember that once a person feels hurt through your interaction that person will try to hurt you back, no matter how innocent your intention may have been. It does not matter if that person is your spouse, your child, your best friend, your co-worker, your brother, your sister, your patient, client, customer, a stranger or even your boss!

As you work towards becoming able to take daily positive action more consistently, be prepared for greater criticisms. **The more you try to be great by doing the best you can, even in the most challenging or hostile circumstances in your life or workplace, the more you shall be challenged to give more or criticized for not doing enough or not doing what others expected. This is the pain of transformation. If you block out the noise and stay focused on your mission, you will transform like a pupa to become a butterfly.**

However, if the noise overwhelms you, the cocoon of other people's opinion will keep you trapped as a pupa. This is sadly one of the reasons why most people give up on trying to become better managers of stress and anxiety in their lives. This is further made worse by a tendency to resort to blaming others when things are not going well.

Unfortunately, this is where most of us make mistakes. We get discouraged and we are not able to make lemonade out of the lemons positively consistent, you will find yourself anxious, sad, depressed and discouraged when you encounter some of the challenges and disappointments of daily life.

One of the biggest sources of stress in your daily life is from your relationships. It may simply be your relationship with your family, friends, or coworkers. One way to reduce this possibility is to ask questions. Asking ourselves these questions and answering them honestly will enable us to enjoy our relationships more fully.

We shall be more prepared for the curved balls that may sometimes come our way in relationships. Sometimes this may mean disappointing your friends and your family. It may mean that you cannot attend as many social events as you would like to. It may even mean saying "No" to yourself. Can you do it? Can you withstand the pressure when the negative comments start trickling in? Can you refuse to participate in the activities you really like so that you can focus on the activities that will help you minimize stress?

Do you know how to cut down on your daily stress outbursts? Do you know the common factors that lead to stress in your daily life? Is it daily criticism?

The impact of criticism on your encounters depends on your perception or attitude. Criticism is one of those inside or outside adverse effects that can disrupt your sense of well-being or homeostasis and lead to recurring daily stress unless you master the skills to manage it . Unless you live all alone and interact with no one, twenty-four hours a day, daily criticisms are inevitable. For most people, criticisms are one of the audiovisual triggers for stress generation. How can you overcome this tendency?

**Don't let those who see only your uncompleted projects and faults, discourage you from believing in yourself and consistently striving to become the better version of yourself in all aspects of your life every day.** If you other people's negative thoughts about you dominate your mind, it can stop you from living a stress-free life, if it makes you focus on the negative instead of on how to improve and achieve more of your goals every day. Don't forget to take action that will help you achieve your work-related goals, social goals, physical, financial, health and wellness and spiritual goals. The more you can take positive action despite the daily criticisms you have to endure, the more you can live a healthier, more positive and longer life!

**Unless you are prepared to acknowledge that every day of your life you will be criticized by others with little or no recognition of your positive attributes, you will not be able to convert the nuggets of daily criticisms into food for your mind and personal transformation.** Remember that through your thoughts and actions you can influence how your brain responds to stress. Dealing with criticism every day can be quite challenging.

Daily stress will become the chronic stress that manifests as loss of concentration, recurrent anxiety, loss of self-confidence and your sense of direction, and even lead to potentially lie-ending conditions like  high blood pressure, asthma, and heart attack. If you want to make your life more stress-free you must learn how to convert relentless criticism into opportunities for becoming a better version of yourself . You can do this by taking action to protect yourself against criticism.

If you get so used to being reminded of your imperfections so much that you begin to believe that you are nothing but the sum of your imperfections, then you will not be able to improve your life. You are not the sum of your imperfections. You're a complex human being with strengths and weaknesses. Sometimes taking action to protect yourself against criticism would entail giving yourself positive self-talk, at other times it would entail becoming charming every day.

Sometimes we get so caught up in our activities of the day that we do not have time to listen intentionally to others. This is unhealthy for our relationships, because when concerns and worries are not shared, emotional tension builds up. This can lead to frustration and anger.

One of the ways to make this work is to cut down on the number of closed conversations we experience with others. How do you do that? Listen with your senses and watch your relationships become more positive.

To really be helpful we must learn to listen with our senses .We have to actively listen with our eyes, ears and even hands. If your hands touch and it is quickly withdrawn, something is wrong. If a hug is rejected something is wrong. A rising and loud voice suggests the buildup of tension. If deliberate avoidance begins to happen, especially if in the past eye contact was freely made, then something is amiss. Ask questions. Make sure you really have what you think you have.

Learn to look at your conversations with others as a chess game. Don't just talk to others without being mentally prepared for how they would respond to you. This could be a negative response from a person that sees problems in everything you do. With others, it could be a positive response. Remember that if you want to win a chess game, you must be able to anticipate 2 or 3 moves your opponent might make after you have made your first move. When you are talking to others, you must form the habit of anticipating responses.

Keep in mind that there may be other factors or other concerns, others may have that affect their dealings with you or could influence their response to you. There could be hidden antagonistic conversational messages in your interactions with others.

Make a note of the number of times your emotional sense of well-being has been disrupted  and you felt stressed out enough to have an outburst during the day. Do this in the morning, the middle of your day and at the end of your day. If you get into stressful outbursts 10 or more times a week , then your compass stress index is more than 100 or more or severe. When it is 5 times to 9 times week, your compass stress index is 50 or more. When it is 0 to 4 times per week, Your Compass Stress Index will be 40 or less.

Your daily objective would be to keep your Compass Stress Index (CSI) to zero per day or one per week.  This means having 1 or less challenging stressful event per week should be your goal. At the end of this course, you would be able to reduce your baseline compass stress index to less than half of what you started with. You will get to a point where every emotional tension will not lead to a stressful outburst. Here is your modified compass stress index(CSI):

Good Compass stress index: 0 to 1stress outburst per week

Mild Compass stress index: 2 to 4 stress outbursts per week

Moderate Compass stress index:5 to 9 stress outbursts per week

Severe Compass stress index: 10 or more stress outbursts per week

Extreme Compass stress index: Any compass stress index with any hostile contact

A compass stress outburst is characterized by yelling, disruptive behavior like pounding or striking things without contact with another person.

Hostile contact with another person in terms shoving, pushing, fighting, or using or brandishing weapons like knives, guns, sticks, stones, glass, regardless of frequency of daily stressful outbursts is an automatic extreme compass stress index that would require immediate action to diffuse the tension and protect your life.

Why? **Extreme compass stress index means DANGER.** What actions will you take when your house is on fire? Do the same when you are dealing or interacting with someone whose behavior has been classified or found to be dangerous or extreme compass stress index. Run for your life!!!

Write down your average compass stress index for the week. The lower the number the better. You should strive for  a weekly compass stress index of zero to one.

Daily evaluation or weekly will help you discover your own trend. Is it going up or going down? **Get a stress-free -living journal or notebook and take notes of the time and circumstances that typically lead to a stress outburst. This will help you discover your own  tendencies, and the commonest causes of stress for you.**

How can you be sure that you are meeting your daily mini goals if you don't evaluate them? Are you regularly having thoughts and conversations that will help you develop consistent positive interactions, so that you can truly and happily be the best version of yourself without fear or favor?

Are you reducing or eliminating those situations that predispose you to stressful interactions? Are you keeping stress out of your relationships and conversations? Do you use gratitude as one of the ways you can manage stress? How can an attitude of gratitude help you to eliminate stress when things go wrong? An attitude of gratitude can help you to eliminate stress in your daily life by helping you change how you think about the situation. Don't forget that the habit of writing the things you are grateful for everyday will help reduce stress, build better relationships, and live a longer and healthier life. What are the three things you are most grateful for today? Do you have a gratitude journal? Start your own gratitude journal today., if you don't already have one.

To become better at managing stress during your interactions with others you have to gain a better understanding of the motivations and personalities that influence your daily interactions. You have to make your daily mini-goals part of your main goal for improving your health and wellness for the week and for the month. If you do this, despite emotional disruptions, obstacles, and challenges, you will end up winning more than losing.

**After you have determined or discovered the easy activities that will consistently help you to eliminate and manage stress, take realistic action to transform yourself and get the results you want for yourself.** Your goals should be achievable and make sense within the parameters of your life. This includes your health, finances, relationships, family, job, education, spirituality, circumstances, situation, thoughts and actions. Be patient with yourself. Be prepared to learn from your own mistakes or from your critics. Don't expect everyone to like or find no fault in what you are doing,

Don't assume because you are now a little bit older others will be more accommodating towards you. Stay vigilant. Even the most beautiful butterfly still gets eaten by a bird! Always stay prepared for the unexpected. Don't assume that because you have spent most of your life taking care of your spouse, children, and parents, that as you begin to get older, one of them will be there for you.

If you always stay  prepared for the unexpected, you will have the right perspective for positive emotional well-being no matter what you are doing or what you are going through. How will you feel if people criticize you after you have given them the best you have to offer. What will you do?

How can you cope when those whom you think should know better criticize you for the very thing in which you give your best? How would you feel if the parents of your students criticized you after you have given your best to your students as a teacher?.

Check your list of activities you consider realistic for you to accomplish your stress-free living  daily objectives in a day based on your knowledge, experience, personality, available resources, and your time – management skills. Once you have a concrete list in front of you, it's a lot easier to check on yourself regularly. You have to stick to your plan and accomplish the tasks on your list one after the other. If you do this day in, day out, week after week, you will gain in your ability manage both the expected and unexpected emotional disruptions and stressful encounters without losing  it back! Do you have the discipline to do your best with what you have every day?

Don't let regular evaluation discourage you, instead use it as a tool to discover either new sources of emotional tension or new wrinkles to old sources of emotional tension, so that you can more effectively manage them and protect your health, sense of well-being and happiness.

Would you rather spend your golden years being a source of wisdom in your family and community, going to the events that you enjoy or spend most of your time in a doctor's waiting room and coming in or out of admissions? You have to remind yourself that staying healthy and being able to do the things you enjoy doing as you get older is less painful and less exhausting than being sick, and spending days and weeks in the hospital.

What is your 30-day stress management challenge? Write down the  most common factors or situations that caused you stress in the past 7 days. What is your biggest challenge or area of frustration or anxiety? What are the most common factors affecting your stress status in the past 7 days? What is your compass stress index(CSI)? Did you reduce your CSI by at least 80% at the end of your 30-day challenge?

# Have more supportive and positive relationships in your life

The sixth key to living a healthier and longer life after 50 is having more supportive and positive relationships. Why are positive and supportive relationships important for living a longer and healthier life? An 85-year Harvard longitudinal research study found that the single most consistent factor for living a longer and healthier life was having positive relationships.

Do you know that you cannot keep positive connections in your relationships without your own daily positive emotional well-being? How can you learn to make the decision to have positive emotional wellness every day? You have to begin by doing a 72- hour relationship audit, to find out the common factors that make your relationships less supportive and positive.

Why does lack of positive and supportive relationships affect our longevity so much? According to the NIH, research has shown that relationship deficits such as social isolation, lack of support, or high strain, can lead to chronic stress and inflammation, which can be bad for your overall health. Becoming better at managing relationship deficits and social isolation is part of the ways you can have more supportive and positive relationships.

Unfortunately, isolation is unfortunately more common as we get older, and can rob you of the positive connections you once had with your spouse, friends, kids, grandkids or even coworkers. Research has shown that poorly managed negative emotions can lead to chronic inflammation which can   affect your cellular and vascular health and  even  your brain health, heart health, liver, kidney, and other organs in your body.

Based on your initial 72-hour health and wellness audit which aspect of your daily interactions with others is the most common or greatest source of emotional disruption in your relationships? What is the most challenging interaction you have had in your relationships? Is it having conversations? Is it asking questions? Is it sharing your own point of view? Relationships are complex and always involve the plain and hidden. They always involve pain and joy. They always include  positive and negative emotions. Research has shown  that those with more positive emotions than negative ones are more resilient and more likely to manage stress better(Fredrickson et al, 2003).

You have to remember that 80% of your disruptions will come from 20% of your encounters?  Reduce your list to the 5 most common encounters with disruptions. Do you know the 1 out of 5 encounters that cause the most disruption to your positive and supportive relationships? How can you always maintain positive interactions in your relationship with others? The key to maintaining positive and supportive relationships in your interactions with others at all times is always to stay prepared for the unexpected.

Relationships can involve you, others, and your environment. While most relationships start with fun and games, overtime, some become filled with trials and tribulations or they simply become boring and predictable. The ability to handle these challenges effectively determines how supportive and fulfilling the relationship will become, and how well you can protect your health, and improve your wellness during such interactions.

**What are positive relationships? Positive relationships are based on mutual trust and respect with value for independence and the understanding that despite our best efforts, sometimes mistakes will be made, or misunderstandings will occur.** In positive relationships each person will be willing to forgive and overlook mistakes without trying to put the other person's feet to the fire.

# 8 Keys To Longevity After 50

By the time you get to 50 years and above, you would have gone through a lot of challenges and disappointments. Maybe you are already divorced or going through a difficult marriage or having challenges with your children or in-laws. One way you can retain your positive emotional wellness and make your relationships more supportive is to forgive yourself and others. Relationships are not the same as mathematics. Sometimes you win by losing. You may be surprised by how simply saying "you are right" may help reduce tension and restore the emotional imbalance in your relationships

Why is forgiveness an important part of a positive and supportive relationship? When you forgive others, you let go of the tension that builds up within you when others annoy you, and let go of the stress, anxiety and resentment that could disrupt your internal milieu. Forgiving is like opening a clinched fist, it helps you to become more receptive to others and to see more possibilities.

The more we are able to forgive without being naïve as we get older, the more inner

---

peace and tranquility we shall enjoy as we get older.

Positive relationships are like team sports, we have to be in it for each other for our team to have the best result. One person in the relay team runs the fastest but if that person does not the baton, the relay team will be disqualified. Being part of a relay team is a commitment. Each member must make the decision to show up or the relay team can't run when it counts the most.

Making the relationships in your daily life positive is also a decision and a commitment to better communication. You have to make the decision to make your relationships more positive. You have to remember that most relationships are based on what people can get out of it. In positive relationships every mistake or something the other person has done differently should not be a 'gotcha moment" or an opportunity for you to judge the other person and tell them how horrible they are.

**Positive relationships are value-adding relationships.** What value do your daily relationships add to your life? What value does person A add to your life? Does your spouse, brother, sister, uncle, auntie add a positive value to your life? Remember that no single person can completely satisfy the needs of another. *Expect to have no more than 80% of your needs fulfilled by your partner, friend or the person you are talking with.* You'll have to find the other 20% somewhere else. This might be the need to watch horror movies with someone else, have intellectual conversations, talk about shopping,  talk about sports or even your spirituality with others with others.

What value do they add to your daily interactions? When you talk to those  close to you do you feel appreciated, valued or do you feel unappreciated and manipulated? Do you feel  judged? Do you feel that you are all still part of a team or is each person now trying to look out only for their own interest, happiness, or enjoyment? Are you interested in a value-driven relationship while your partner is interested in a benefit-driven relationship? It is difficult to have a positive relationship in a cocoon of negativity.

**Another way to make your relationships more positive is to manage your expectations. What are your expectations when you communicate with others? Can you deal with the criticisms and conflicts that are part and parcel of daily communication?** If you want to maintain your own peace of mind throughout the day, then you have to be prepared for unmet expectations. Sometimes it will come in the form of others not wanting to talk when you want to talk. Sometimes, it will come in the form of others disagreeing with you or calling you names even when you thought you were doing your best and acting in the best interest of everyone. What will you do?

You have to remember that as long as the someone  feels that what you have done or are doing is not right or fair, that  person will get a negative emotional response from you or from whatever you say. That person may be your son, daughter, mom, father, friend or co-worker. Sometimes the response will be subtle and mild, at other times it will be a moderate or even a severe repudiation of you as a person and what you purportedly stand for or believe in. You might even be mocked or called a hypocrite or failure. If you were already mentally prepared for any outcome, you won't really be too surprised by what others say. To foresee is to rule!

If you are the head of the family, the manager, the lead, the director, or boss, be prepared to be blamed more than others. Don't assume that others will understand when you explain to them why you are struggling or why things are not quite going as planned. Focus on finding your own peace through gratitude and positive thinking, rather hoping to be understood and appreciated.

People are surprised when they have emotional problems in their relationships. This is because most people think that because they have married someone they deeply love, everything would be wonderful. This is a false belief. Every relationship has its beautiful moments and challenging moments. This is why it is important to make your emotional expectations realistic. Don't expect others to be kind to you or speak kindly about you when they are upset with you.

According to the NIH, psychoneuroimmunology has found that there is a relationship between negative emotions and inflammation. Chronic inflammation leads to poor long-term health (Renna, 2021). One of the keys to effective self-mastery is the ability to embrace your difficulties and challenges. Instead of trying to completely figure out how you can avoid criticisms by doing everything within your power to become compliant with another person's sense of what is right or wrong, focus on the strategies that will help you convert daily criticisms into stress-free encounters by turning them into opportunities for greater improvement and more healthy living.

**What would you do in that circumstance? Will you try to explain what happened and what you think led to the**

**misunderstanding? Will you keep quiet and remind yourself that explanations explain nothing? By answering the above questions, you will have a better understanding of the plain and  hidden factors affecting your relationships with others. Nobody is everything the other person expected.** Nobody is perfect!

Avoid the belief that a good relationship is good 100% of the time. It is not true and creates unreasonable expectations. It is like expecting perfection from others when you know that no one is perfect. Expect that challenges will occur and be prepared for them. Your health and wellness depend on it!!  Make your expectations more realistic. No one person gives 100 percent all the time. Why is it that even when you do not give 100% all the time you expect 100% from others?

Make the decision not to let the negative things people will say about you when things don't go as expected or they don't get what they wanted from your interaction with you, pull down your spirit or make you doubt yourself. Try your best not to bear grudges particularly when you feel that though you were trying to be the best version of yourself in a given moment or situation, another person saw you as the worst person ever from their own perspective and  perception of that same moment or situation.

Before you know the other person well or interacted with them in a myriad of situations and circumstances, it's easy to imagine they're everything you'd ever need from another person: a soul mate, sounding board, best friend, the perfect gentleman, lady, or perfect lover.

When the urge to do something different comes, will you  ignore it or justify your inaction through a list of excuses and reasons. These will range from lack of time, to lack of money, to fear of failure or fear of disrupting family and social commitments. In the end you will find yourself in the category of people who know the type of life they would really like to be living but settle for less. Forming habits that will help you achieve greater balance in your life and improve your health by living an intentional life is part of your holistic self-mastery.

The third way is to deal with related **trust issues.** Do you have trust-related issues in your life? Some people have difficulty trusting others. Some people are more resentful than others when they don't receive the level of trust, they think they deserve or the praise they think deserve in their relationships. Be trustworthy and expect the same from your partner. There are little things you can do to build trust, keep your word. Be on time, be open, don't be jealous Don't lie about what you have done or your whereabouts.

The other  way is to be prepared to manage financial **disagreements.** Financial issues often lead to relationship challenges. It's easy for the feelings of stress and anxiety to be taken out on your partner. Don't assume that the more money you have, the more others will love you and listen to you. You have to blame someone, right? Don't. Build up a team with your partner to deal with financial challenges and other challenges.

Remember that even those that you love can resent you. Keep everyone involved, otherwise, one person will deal with challenges and feelings of resentment. Believe me! Resentment is not good for your health. A resentment-filled relationship is not a supportive and healthy relationship. You need to learn to identify the common sources of resentment in your relationships and avoid them.

At home or with the family, resentment sometimes comes from the feeling that only one person is doing most of the work or that things are not fair. It could be the sense that one person is doing most of the chores at home, while the other person is not keeping to an agreed division of labor. Who does the dishes every night? Who cooks every day? Who makes the money for the family? Who makes the decisions in the family?

How can you keep positive relationships at home, work, and social surroundings? At home do you have a list of family daily chores? Make one! Make a list of all the chores that need to be done. Divide them into three lists – daily, weekly, and monthly. You might consider taking turns choosing chores. After a few months, you can swap. At work and at social gatherings make sure you accord everyone their respect and dignity. Don't let the titles that people have befuddle you.

**The sixth way to make your relationship healthier is to make sure you don't destroy your relationships by cheating or telling lies. While the urge to cheat may be real, you have to remember that once you cheat you destroy trust in your relationship.** Without trust your relationship becomes unhealthy and filled with doubt, stress, and anxiety. Dealing with stress and anxiety every day will make you more prone to chronic inflammation and the related chronic diseases like high blood pressure, auto immune disease, depression, and inflammatory bowel disease.

How do you know that your spouse is really working late when he says he is working late? How do you know that a business trip to New York was not really been a weekend gateway with a lover in Hawaii?  Cheating is the result of short-term thinking and will destroy your health and wellness unless you keep your eye on the long-term benefits of a healthy relationship.

When there is nothing to look forward to, the relationship stops growing. You need to set a few goals together to make the future more interesting and plan trips, projects or reasonable big purchases together. Get out of the house at least once a week, at the most once a month for an event together. Look for ways to make your relationship more supportive. It could be eating out, going to the movies or a sporting event together, or going for a walk together. yoga class, or bowling.

If you use these ways in your relationships, you will make them more resilient, and positive and less dominated by stress and anxiety. Though having a positive and supportive relationships can help you cut down on chronic stress and help you to live a more intentional life, it is still good to know the common causes of criticisms and conflicts in your daily attempts at having more positive and supportive relationships.

Did you know that daily criticism is one of the factors that can rob you of your positive emotional wellbeing and positive relationships? Your health and well-being can easily be overrun by daily criticisms. Daily criticism can become one of the factors that can rob you of your positive emotions and disrupt your focus on intentional living.

Research has shown that maintaining positive emotions like  gratitude, pride, joy, interest, hope, inspiration, and contentment will help you to learn how to overcome the weed of daily criticism in your garden of life.

Where do the criticisms and complaints about you occur the most?  Do they criticisms occur at home or only at work or during social interactions able to find out the common causes of criticisms in your life, do some additional analysis to find out the 1 out of 5 triggers of criticisms in your life that generates 80% of your criticisms? Once you learn to manage the 20% source of 80% of your daily criticisms, you will find yourself having greater peace of mind and good health.

Research has shown that criticism makes the one being criticized mentally exhausted, have low esteem, lose confidence, get depressed, anxious, and become more prone to self-harm. The more you are criticized, the more you want to resist or want to do anything at all. Sadly, for those who criticize you, not wanting to do anything further justifies their criticism.

How would you feel if you find yourself in a situation where you are always being corrected or reminded of your faults and inadequacies without any acknowledgement of your positive attributes or positive contributions to your relationship or interactions with others? Most people find such situations unbearable!

The problem is that those that criticize have a need to be correct and make others do things differently. In their mind they think they are helping you improve, but the reality is that the person who is being criticized could find such behavior totally negative. Negativity eventually erodes the foundation of your wellness, positive emotional well-being, and more supportive relationships.

One of the ways you can create more positive and supportive relationships is to help yourself have a positive warrior mindset. Self–assertiveness will help you to support your position with facts while being mindful of the other person's feelings and perspective.

When it comes to daily communications, it is important to pay particular attention to how you relate to your family, friends, and co-workers. Though your family may love you and genuinely want the best for you, you still have to take daily action to get the best out of your life. This is because family members can be brutally critical of your efforts when the results, they get out of your efforts do need meet their emotional and financial needs. Use your self-talk to prepare yourself for the unexpected. Stick to your healthy living goals even if they are not universally approved.

The bottom line is that whether you are dealing with friends, families, or co-workers, it is important to make sure you understand the full meaning of your conversations with them. If you are not able to do this, you will find yourself constantly having misunderstandings and shouting matches with your friends and loved ones. This will lead to daily anxiety, criticisms, frustrations, and stress that can drain your energy and ultimately diminish your ability to live a healthy, long, and intentional life! your thought process and make your communication more effective.

If you change your way of thinking, you will change your life and overcome the fear of failure which can stop you from trying your best to in all your dimensions of wellness. Picture yourself winning in those scenarios and think deeply about how you would feel after you have formed the sustainable habits that will help you live healthy.

**Celebrate small victories along the way but be prepared for unexpected setbacks.** Having small victories as you pursue your ultimate dream will train you for greater success.

**Not everyone will be happy to see that you have not given up on your dreams or that you refuse to let the fear of failure stop you from trying to be your best in all aspects of daily your life.** If you stay focused and refuse to let what others think about you determine how you feel, you will eventually get most of what you want from your daily opportunities.

Don't let your day be full of missed opportunities. Learn to see the possibility for weight loss in every encounter or event that makes up your day. You can do this by directing your energy into making the most out of your daily situations instead of trying to determine whom to blame or whom to chastise. Focus on taking advantage of your daily opportunities rather than on the words and actions of those who generate a lot of negative energy with little or no capacity to support your goals.

You must learn to minimize the tendency to think of the worst outcomes all the time. **Rather than thinking the worst about a situation or an event, remind yourself that remaining positive through difficult times will help you to transform your daily reality. This type of focus will help you to continue to stay healthy even if all those around you think that you can't.**

If you do not invest in yourself and in your ability to find out new and better ways to make the most out of your daily opportunities, your dreams and goals will remain illusions to be pursued but ultimately unrealized. You can avoid such an outcome by learning how to spot opportunities and consistently take positive action to transform your opportunities into accomplishments.

Unfortunately, some of these negative reactions may include giving up on the actions that can help you make your relationships more positive and supportive. Remind yourself that when you remember the things you are grateful for when the going gets tough will help you to become more positive. It is challenging to keep an attitude of gratitude when things are not going as expected at home, at work or during your daily interactions with others. This is particularly true if you have tried to be the best version of yourself in all aspects of your life and have fallen short. This typically leads to frustration and anger, and people sometimes lash out. Don't lash out at yourself or others, remember that with gratitude "you can turn your problems into gifts, and failures into success".

You have to learn how to focus on an attitude of gratitude even when you think you are not being treated fairly! This is hard because the natural tendency is to lash out in anger when others annoy you or get disappointing results. Simply put, you want to counterattack!

Instead of going on the attack, learn how to have an attitude of gratitude, so that you can be  more strategic in your response. Be open to the many lessons that life will teach you. Instead of resenting such lessons, you should embrace them and see them as opportunities for keeping your peace in the midst of the storms or challenges of daily life as  you get older. Remember that by the time you get to 50 years and above, you have probably lived more than half of your life.

You have to remember that one of the best ways to keep an attitude of gratitude is to try to work hard at accomplishing your daily tasks.  If you stop worrying about outcomes and focus on giving your best effort in every situation you find yourself,   you will positively  feel  more  fulfilled  and  less stressed out. Gratitude will help you to engender positive emotions which will help you reduce chronic inflammation and improve your health. According to NIH, an attitude of gratitude is associated with better mood  and  sleep,  less  fatigue,  more  self-efficacy, and a lower cellular inflammatory index (Mills et al, 2015).

The simplest way to do this regularly is to remind yourself of the reasons why you are grateful. You could be grateful that you are healthy and do not have to deal with a life-changing illness that could prevent you from working and earning the livelihood that allows you and your family to live the lifestyle that you have. You could even be grateful for the simple reason that when you were rushing to work today, you narrowly missed hitting a pedestrian at the crosswalk. Did you know that an attitude of gratitude can help you deal better with situations such as having diabetes, high blood pressure, COPD, heart failure or COVID 19 or financial challenges?

You need to have the mental energy to make the right decisions and take the actions that will reflect your values and priorities while saying no to distractions and wrong priorities when dealing with others and pursuing your goal of living longer.

Have you formed the habits that will help you pursue and achieve your daily goals?

Everyone has habits. They are either having a positive effect on you or a negative one.

A habit can also be defined or described as a behavior that is recurrent, that is acquired or formed through repeated action that is usually brought on by a cue or social context (Rubin, 2015). Research has shown that about 40 % to 50% of our daily activities are shaped by habits. Do you know the habits that dominate your own daily activities? Are you an early riser? Do you get your projects done right away or at the last minute? Do you like to get things done step by step or on the fly? Do you easily get distracted, or do you begin one project before you start another?

As you try to form the good habits that will help you in your pursuit of your purpose in life, some people around you will tell you to give up your dreams and settle for the familiar and the usual. What will you do? You can use positive self-talk to change your life. According to Dr Caprio and Joseph Berger, we can overcome nervous tension, fatigue, insomnia and use our dreams to have a better life by directing our subconscious mind to change our habits and attitudes through positive self-talk. Some people consider positive self-talk to be the autosuggestion step in self-hypnosis.

You will totally enjoy doing things that you are passionate about. Setbacks, difficulties, and obstacles will make it more challenging, but should not deter you from pursuing your goals. Naturally, there may be barriers that may prevent you from reaching your goal, but your heart's desire will find ways to overcome these barriers so that you may ultimately live a healthier, longer, and more fulfilled life.

What is your 30-day positive-warrior mindset challenge? Get your guided longevity journal to keep track of your positive mind set use or lack of., when you have been angry. Out of 30 days, did you meet your goals at least 80% of the time.

# Form the habit of living with  a positive warrior mindset

A positive warrior mindset is the seventh to living a longer life. Why is a positive mindset one of the keys to living a healthier, longer and happier life?  While we cannot control the problems we will encounter in our daily lives, we can control how we can react to them through our positive warrior mindset.

Can you commit to consistently taking small positive steps every day? Are prepared for the fact that you always have to deal with problems every day? What are you doing with the numerous thoughts that stream into your mind every day?

If you find yourself focusing on the mistake you made at the beginning of your day, or only on the mistakes you have made during your day, then you are not looking enough at things through  the perspective of a positive warrior mind set or growth mindset. You have a negative self-talk. If you acknowledge the negative while trying to figure out how to get the most positive out of a challenging situation you have a positive self-talk and a positive warrior mind set.

As you get older you have to deal with the potential problems with your health like high blood pressure, diabetes, heart disease, weight-related problems or even cancer. You also have to deal with potential problems with your job, retirement concerns, financial concerns, your relationship with your children, spouse, siblings and parents. What will you do?

Write down a list of your activities and actions in the past 72 hours of your life and see the situations and circumstances that predominantly made you look at things negatively. These are the types of negative patterns that can lead to chronic negative feelings, emotional tension, poor emotional control, stress, and unhappiness, that you need to learn how to use your positive warrior mind set or positive self-talk to manage better.

A study  from John Hopkins found that those with family history of heart disease and also had a positive outlook were about 33% less likely to have a heart attack or related cardiovascular event in 5 to 25 years than those  who had a negative mindset or outlook. When your mind becomes overwhelmed by negativity you lose the ability  to look at things positively. You lose the ability to look at things with a positive mind set. One of the best ways you can use the positive warrior mindset would be to consistently stay positive in everything you need to do every day. Does that mean that you will succeed in everything you do every day? No. It means you will continue to try until you succeed in your own way. Cut down on distractions and participation in activities that don't help you to live a happy, healthier, and longer life.

You have to remember that the way you communicate with yourself will significantly affect the outcome of anything you do.

According to Marcus Aurelius, "The happiness of your life depends on the quality of your thoughts." Do you know what is affecting your confidence in yourself and your ability to make healthy decisions? Is it what others will say? Is it your inability to say, "No" to others when they encourage to eat or drink something that you would normally try? What is holding you back from making a commitment to living a more healthy and more positive life? Is it fear of the process or fear of communication with others? Is it the fear of failure?

You have to begin where you are then make adjustments as you go along. Make sure you use your positive warrior mindset or growth mindset to make the right decisions in your life. Some people make the wrong decision and drink so much alcohol that they lose control of their mind and end up getting involved in fights, drunk driving, or toxic sexual behavior. Sometimes such behavior can lead to the death of innocent bystanders.

What use will eating healthy food, exercising every day be to you, if you drink so much alcohol that you crash and kill yourself? This is an example of poor self-care and failed sociocultural, emotional, and physical wellness.   Remember that the lowest common wellness pathway and for emotional wellness, it is listening more and speaking less.

Are you making a positive difference in your life and in the life of others? You can make a positive difference in your life and What is the pattern of thinking that dominates how you handle your daily activities, problems and challenges? Do you have a negative or positive pattern of thinking?  Your negative pattern of thinking can cloud your thoughts and rob you of the clarity that you need to make outcome-driven decisions. Unless you learn how to change this pattern of thinking, you will find yourself giving up on your opportunity to learn from your mistakes, become a better person and live a healthier, happier and longer life.

Make your conversations with others focus more on describing problems and offering solutions rather on evaluating  others and telling them about the things they have done wrong and their negative traits, lack of congruence and lack of sincerity. Unfortunately, most of us love to tell others what they have done wrong.

Do you know that communication is an important part of a positive warrior mindset? Do you remember that the "C" in the compass profile represents community relationships and communications? Research shows that supportive communication means a more problem-oriented rather than person-oriented communication.

While it is true that we need to always be prepared to face problems in life, we also need to learn  how to manage daily problems through our thoughts and actions. This means you focus on events and behaviors rather than on personal inadequacies and traits. If you are dealing with a difficult person or someone who is usually quick to judge or very negative in outlook be prepared to bend without breaking. Don't call such a person names or say things like, "you are wicked", you are difficult", "you are always unfair", such words or sentences will make people undervalued and unappreciated. When people feel bad about themselves, they tend to strike back in anger.

People don't take negative interactions well. It will take positive self-talk to learn not to take negative comments personally. Even if someone falsely accuses you, calls you names or tells you, you are wicked, stay calm. Think of the outcome of what you are about to say before you say it. If it would lead to emotional imbalance and negatively affect your mood and what you eat, don't say it.

Do you know that feelings of gratitude can contribute to your positive warrior mindset? Are you living with gratitude? What are you grateful for today? Form the habit of starting and ending each day by stating the 3 things you are most grateful for. This is a very important activity that you must start and do every day. This is a simple life transforming habit that can help you put things in perspective and have peace that no one can take away from you.

Don't forget that even if you start your day with one problem, it does not mean that your whole day will be bad. That problem may actually turn out to be a blessing in disguise if you tackle it with patience and integrity.

The more you know about yourself, the easier it will be for you to discover what you really want in life and make a concerted effort to pursue it. Sadly, most of us do not know what we really want in life until it's time to die – and that's a shame. The challenge most of us have is that we find it difficult to narrow our focus.

According to Bussing et al, ..feelings of gratitude and awe contribute to positive perceptions and cognitions even in the face of illness and disease. Research has also shown that higher levels of gratitude are directly linked to better social support and reduction in stress and depression(Wood et al., 2008).

Remind yourself of 3 things you are grateful for when the going gets tough. It is challenging to keep an attitude of gratitude when things are not going as expected at home, at work or during your daily interactions with others. This is particularly true if you have tried to be the best version of yourself in all aspects of your life and have fallen short. This typically leads to frustration and anger, and people sometimes lash out. Don't lash out at yourself or others, remember that with gratitude "you can turn your  problems into gifts, and failures into success".

The simplest way to do this regularly is to remind yourself of the reasons why you are grateful. You could be grateful that you are healthy and do not have to deal with a life-changing illness that could prevent you from working and earning the livelihood that allows you and your family to live the lifestyle that you have. You could even be grateful for the simple reason that when you were rushing to work today, you narrowly missed hitting a pedestrian at the crosswalk. Did you know that an attitude of gratitude can help you deal better with situations such as having diabetes, high blood pressure, COPD, heart failure or COVID 19 or financial challenges?

However, if you focus on "how", you will be able to start thinking of how to solve the problem or deal with the situation. While it is good to find out why you are not getting the result you expected from your interactions with others, finding out how you can get better results will help you think more clearly and strategize more effectively. Doing this will help you change your attitude from fear and apprehension and help you take action for solution-oriented achievable results (SOAR).

**Everyone makes mistakes but only great minds learn how to minimize them and**

**get better results, rather than wallowing in explanations and recriminations. You too can become a great mind!**

Does that mean that we should focus on positive things and deny negative emotions? No. A habit of gratitude does not mean that we ignore complicated feelings, difficult decisions, and challenging experiences (Amanda Breon, 2021). It just means that we do not dwell on the negative, without focusing on  finding the positive in the negative.

For some people, revealing themselves to others makes them become more critical and more fault-finding. They then begin to condemn their friends, loved ones and co-workers for everything. This may range from telling people that they are  barely good at their jobs  to telling them that they are grossly incompetent. This is a dangerous spiral because this is part of an evaluative and person-oriented communication that leads to hurt on both sides.

Strategic thinking is very important because it will help you become more intentional. What is strategic thinking? Think about outcome and impact before you speak and act? It will also help you to focus more on those activities that will enable you to accomplish your goals rather on emotional flexing to make you feel good and put the other person in his or her place. **Go the extra mile in finishing your tasks.**
**Without consistent implementation your goals will remain illusions**. Try taking risks but never compromise your safety. Taking risks means that you are ready to learn new things and tackle challenges that will help you continue to grow as a person. **A warrior mindset is very important in achieving your goals.** You do not allow your obstacles and setbacks to define you.

How can you cope when those whom you think should know better criticize you for the very thing in which you give your best?

How would you feel if parents criticized you after you have given your best to your students as a teacher? How will you feel if people criticize you after you have given them the best you have to offer. What will you do?

You have to remember that just because you have told the truth or because you believe you are acting for the common good does not mean everyone will accept it. You may still be called a liar despite your best efforts to be fair and balanced.

**Don't take disappointments, rejections, or strong opinions personally. If you focus on the love you have for yourself, you will help yourself heal emotionally when you have to deal with a hostile encounter**. You have to remind yourself that one of the keys to healthy living is focusing on what you can control. You can control your ability to try to the  best version of yourself in everything you do, but you cannot control how people will interpret it or react to your efforts.

---

Don't let name calling make you more anxious and less confident. **It depends on how the truth will affect the other person's interest and emotions. This is one of the reasons why thinking more positively about yourself every day is crucial to your ability to manage daily emotions better.**

Most of us find it hard to manage our emotions on a day-to-day basis. Our emotional well-being is very important for our health, well-being and  relationships because feeling good about ourselves reduces our daily stress level and helps to make our interactions with others more enjoyable and fulfilling.

This is important because on any given day you can go through a range of emotions from happiness to sadness, from anger to joy, from elation to disappointment. How can you better manage your emotions so that your relationships will be more enjoyable? **You have to focus on getting a positive emotional outcome out of every encounter you have with others despite spoken and**

**unspoken criticisms.** This is not easy because criticisms or personal attacks during interactions with loved ones, friends or co-workers can become painful emotional wounds. To deal with these types of negative interactions, outbursts, or attacks, remind yourself that every opinion is not an automatic reflection of the truth.

Our emotions or feelings help us to relate to ourselves and to others. This is why any change in our emotional well-being can have a very serious impact on our relationships. It can very easily lead to fights and physical abuse. This is why we need to find and learn new ways to manage our emotions. You can make the decision to have positive emotional wellness throughout your daily encounters and interactions with others.

Just because your emotions feel right does not mean you have a right to scream at others. Be honest with your feelings but make sure you also accept other people's expression of their own feelings.

The important emotional balance approach is to understand the types of events that lead to emotional breakdowns and take steps to overcome them. Most disruptions in emotion usually start with a rise in emotional tension. Once this tension has been recognized, you need to deflect this tension build up through better communication. Sometimes this may entail changing the subject or simply keeping quiet.

Relationships are not the same as mathematics. Sometimes you win by losing. You may be surprised how simply saying "you are right" may help reduce tension and restore the emotional balance in your relationships.

Whatever method you eventually decide to use to manage your emotions remember that even your best may not always be good enough. Sometimes you have to be grateful for the opportunity to have tried. You can't win all the time. You cannot always get the results that you want, diffuse tension by asking yourself to list at least 3 things you are thankful for in the last 72 hours.

An attitude of gratitude will help you learn to use your conversations to overcome daily stress, even when things are not going as well as expected.  If you learn to speak with empathy and seek to build up the self-esteem of all those you deal with at work, at home, or other events, you will find yourself less stressed-out and more effective. You have to do this by being aware of non-verbal cues, supporting your positions with facts and being willing to acknowledge that mistakes can be made despite your best efforts.  Do you see problems as opportunities for growth or hassles that drain your energy?

When dealing with the different circumstances and situations you encounter in your daily life, make sure you stay focused on being the best you can be in the moment of encounter. This is not as easy as it appears because it is easy to get angry when others disrespect you and see nothing good in anything that you do.

Don't let them discourage you. Acknowledge and determine the source and cause of your anger. A strong emotion has to be acknowledged before it can be resolved. If someone or something is making you angry, admit it. Unresolved anger escalates, and your bitterness will show in your interaction with other people. Diffuse anger and it will relieve the stress in your system

Focus on yourself and the steps you need to take every day to help you stay more positive as you deal with the situation and circumstances you find yourself in. Remember that "Your present circumstances don't determine where you can go; they merely determine where you start." Nido Qubein  Remember that a positive mindset can help you find hope even in the most challenging situations and circumstances.

What kind of mindset are  you using in your approach to the different challenges in your daily life? According to Carol Dweck, a renowned psychologist, a fixed mindset person believes that his or her basic

---

qualities, like talent and intelligence, are fixed and cannot be improved. A person with a fixed mindset loves conspiracy theories and external explanations and manipulations for everything that is going on in their lives. On the other hand, a person with a growth mindset or warrior mindset believes that qualities like talent and intelligence can be improved. Stop trying to succeed through short cuts, it will only lead to half measures and failure.

Can you commit yourself to unlimited positive action despite numerous challenges and disappointments? Can you commit to consistently taking small positive steps every day? You can do this by developing a growth mindset. According to Carol Dweck, a renowned psychologist, a fixed mindset person believes that his or her basic qualities, like talent and intelligence, are fixed and cannot be improved. A person with a growth mindset believes that qualities like talent and intelligence can be improved. Fixed mindset people believe that talent alone creates success without effort. It is like believing that you are either born great or you are not.

Research has shown that those with a growth mindset know that through the application of different strategies they can improve. If you do not already have a growth mindset, get one. You can change from a fixed mindset to a growth mindset. One of the best ways you can use the growth mindset would be to consistently pursue excellence in different aspects of your life through commitment to unlimited positive daily action. You can do this through strategy, effort, process, and persistence (SEPP). You can either develop your own SEPP (Strategy, Effort, Process and Persistence) or add more to the one you have already developed. The other one is finding out what motivates you. Do you have a unifying motivational thread throughout all these changes? Many people will turn to their faith or religious beliefs to help them uncover their unifying motivation. limited understanding of yourself. You have to learn to be patient with yourself when trying to get a better understanding of yourself. This is because according to Benjamin Franklin, an inventor and one of the founding fathers of America, to know one's self is as hard as steel or diamond.

Daily good habits are the tools through which you can act on your motivations every day. When you form the habits that will help you stay focused on taking consistent daily action to achieve your goals, instead of complaining and lamenting on your daily setbacks, you shall be well on your way to living a great life. Are you prepared to form the habits that will help you to live a healthier and longer life?
You need to start thinking in a more positive way, learn to look on the bright side and stop being so negative. Research has shown that those with a growth mindset know that through the application of different strategies, like getting input from others, reading, and persistence in action, they can improve and change from average to better.

Form the habit of looking for strategic solutions to problems instead of complaining. The more time you spend complaining the less you will get done. There is a saying that those who complain remain in the same place. Instead of complaining start taking action. Act on your ideas. Don't let the perfect become the enemy of the possible. Wasting time or doing the wrong thing at the wrong time is a reflection of  a negative mindset that is dominated by fear and procrastination

Beginning early is part of the process of using time wisely. This process can help you live a better and more positive life. Remember that one of the keys to  having a positive warrior mindset is the ability to consistently make the right adjustments when the unexpected happens. You have to learn to use your mind to make your goals steppingstones towards living a better life. Ask for help or look for strategic partnerships. Some goals may even lead to conflicts that might make you think of giving up on your ambitions and dreams. Take heart. Consider it an opportunity for collaboration. Remember that goal setting is focused on your benefits. Remind yourself of the benefits of your actions and activities as you try working things out.

Remember that to foresee is to rule. A situation that requires a solution can be approached in a variety of ways. Everyone is free to interpret this in his or her own unique way. Any interpretation by itself is creativity at work. A person who enjoys creative thinking can easily come up with innovative solutions for situations that require a quick fix. However, don't assume that because you like creative ways to solve problems, everyone will support your ideas. Expect the unexpected. If you want to do this consistently, you have to develop the mental discipline that will help you not to complain, when the unexpected happens or when problems prop up in your daily life. Make it a habit to A Bridge Across The Atlantic, "Improvement never ends". You have to make striving to improve part of your daily creative strategy for trying to have a positive warrior mindset.

What is your positive and supportive relationship 30-day challenge? How many

---

times in the past 7 days did you look at problems from a solution perspective than from a blame perspective? How many times were you able to neutralize your negative tendencies in your relationships through positive self-talk in the past 30 days? You need to get to being able to have more positivity from your interactions at least 80% of the time.

## Pay attention to your holistic self-care every day

Paying attention to your holistic self-care is the eighth key to longevity. How can you improve yourself and your self-care today, if you have no idea of how to control the factors that could influence your health? Are you in control of your health, finances, goals, your emotions, relationships, spirituality, time management, environmental, sexual, and social activities?

Are you cautious and careful? What do you think will happen to you if you exercised every day, ate healthy, slept well but didn't pay attention to falls and accidents? This simply shows that you are not paying attention to your holistic self-care. Why is this important? According to research the top three preventable injury-related death in the United States are poisoning, motor vehicles, and falls.

Did you do a periodic gap analysis in your life to discover those areas in your life and environment that need improvement? Are you in a toxic relationship? Are you in a value adding or value subtracting relationship? Are you actively participating in your own journey of health and wellness journey?

While it is important to improve your health and live longer by doing most of the things that I have shared with  so far in this book or training, it is still possible for us to inadvertently cut our lives short by failing to take simple steps that can help us protect our lives through holistic self-care.

A few years ago, there was the tragic story of 78-year-old man in Los Angeles who tragically fell into the pool in his son's house and died. The saddest part of the story was that the son had invited his father over to spend the week there, so that he could spend more time with his grand kids. While this particular fall led to drowning,  at other times falls among those 65 years and above have led to hip fractures, broken necks, spinal and head injuries.

*Protect your home from falls and accidents.

Part of holistic self-care is paying attention to details. For others  the problem is not falls, but motor vehicle accidents. One of the challenges with accidents is that sometimes you may be in a hurry for other reasons then find yourself driving too fast. What if you had started your morning with a drink of fruit smoothies, done your morning exercise and meditation but because you were running late to work or a meeting you forgot to put on your seat belt, and while driving too fast ended up in an accident? Will this be a good outcome for your longer life?

Do you know the most common factors that can affect your holistic self-care? Do your own 72-hour audit to get an idea. Some of the factors that can affect your holistic self-care would include the falls and accidents already mentioned above and other factors that include personal habits and community relationships.

The important thing about improving your holistic self-care is that it helps you to look at the factors that can affect your health and longevity as part of the same continuum. If you ignore one part of the whole, it could lead to deadly and unexpected consequences. You must always stay prepared for unexpected life challenges.

Keep an eye on yourself through the regular use of health and wellness journals. Sometimes part of your immediate self-care would mean ignoring a driver that cut you off though you had right of way. People generally don't like letting go when other drivers cut them off or do something they consider unacceptable. Managing anger has to be part of your holistic self-care because uncontrolled anger could lead to immediate road rage, deadly fights or shoot outs. Is someone cutting you off worth dying for?

Sometimes better immediate self-care will mean ignoring a group of bikers that gave you the middle finger because they didn't like the way you were driving. At other times, it is the other way, it is the bikers putting up with nonsense driving from car drivers. Either way don't retaliate, hold your fire! Remember every action will lead to a reaction. Learn to take chess actions. Think about two of three reactions before you take your first action, and ask yourself if your first is worth it or not?

Your holistic self-care also involves your environment and how you interact with it. A few years ago, a 27-year-old healthy young woman went to the Grand Canyon, and in attempt to take a selfie, slipped off the edge and fell to her death. This is an example of not paying close attention to your surroundings and environment at all times. Paying attention to your surroundings and your environment is part of your immediate holistic self-care.

Have you formed the habit of paying attention to your surroundings and environment? Don't forget that Brutus betrayed Cesar. Be careful with the kind of friends that you hang out with. Some friends will try to get you drunk, poison you or fail to warn you when they see a life-threatening danger coming your way. To foresee is to rule.

Apart from these immediate factors that could put your life in danger you can't ignore your medium to long-term self-care. Don't ignore going for  your yearly physical or doing your recommended screening tests because of your age or family circumstance or history because you are busy or don't really feel like it. Don't ignore or dismiss nagging or persistent symptoms without proper checkup because this could be the difference between discovering cancer at an early stage or at an advanced stage.

 *Keep your appointment with your healthcare providers.

*Do your yearly physical.

*Do your screening tests as recommended by your doctor or healthcare providers.

.*Check and maintain your health insurance.

Do you know that taking your daily vitamins can be part of daily self-care? Do you know that regularly taking vitamins every day is one of the ways you can improve your self-care? Take your daily supplements but do not let them replace your healthy habits and do not forget to let your physician know that you are taking vitamins and supplements.

For example, take your omega 3 and 6 fatty acids which have been proven to be very helpful for the heart. However, do not give up on fish just because you take Omega fatty acids. Still stick to the habit of eating fish rich in Omega fatty acids at least once a week.

According to Wen-Ben Chiou, Ph.D., a professor at Sun Yat-Sen University, "taking dietary supplements increases perceived invulnerability." He reported this in a study in psychological science. Make sure you talk to your doctor about any supplements you are taking or plan to take. This is because if there are interactions or potential interactions between your supplements and any medication you are taking your doctor will let you know. Taking your supplements should not stop you from going for your regular medical checkup as recommended for your age group and family history by your doctor or health care provider.

Apart from supporting heart health, Omega 3 is also good for brain health because research has shown that omega-3 fatty acids help to build cell membranes in the brain. You can get Omega 3 fatty acids from supplements or from fish. This is one of the reasons why it is recommended that you eat fish at least once a week. Begin by making the decision to eat fish at least once a week, you will help your brain health and memory as you get older.

Remind yourself that you are trying to protect your brain health and prevent yourself from getting dementia and preserve your cognitive functions such as attention, learning, thinking, problem solving, decision making, and memory for as long as you can as you get older. The more you preserve your cognitive functions and memory as you get older, the less mistakes, accidents and falls you are likely to have  as you get older.

Eating more fish in your meals will help to get more of the EPA and DHA omega fatty acids that will protect your cells and fight off inflammation and preserve your brain health and the health of your other organs. Keep in mind that it is not a magic wand for all your problems.

It is a huge mistake to assume that simply because you use multivitamins you will remain perfectly healthy or suffer only mild illness. Remember that vitamins are usually supplemental and your taking daily multivitamins will be most effective only if you continue to eat healthy, exercise regularly and continue to manage your weight and the sources of daily stress in your life.

For example, we know that vitamin B can be found in fish, meat, orange juice and fortified cereals, yet we also know we do not always get to eat enough of the food types I have just listed. If you combine trying to eat right with taking your vitamins, you will end up regularly getting enough vitamin B in your body. This is an example of how you can use vitamins as a health supplement.

Why are B vitamins so important? Because they help to lower the level of homocysteine in blood vessels, which at high levels can lead to damage of the lining of arteries and could lead to a faster formation of blood clots.

Are you getting  enough magnesium into your system? How does magnesium affect your health and wellness? Research has shown that magnesium can help to protect your brain health, help you sleep better and lower your blood pressure. What is the best way of getting your daily magnesium?

How much magnesium is recommended daily? For women the recommended daily amount of magnesium is 320 mg and for men, 420mg. A common and easily available source of magnesium is banana. Instead of relying on a single fruit to get your daily magnesium, it may be better to include other foods and fruits like avocado, leafy green vegetables, and nuts like almonds, cashew nuts and peanuts. Other sources of magnesium include chia seeds, pumpkin seeds, brown rice, and black beans.

When you find that you cannot get enough magnesium from your daily meals, consider adding magnesium supplements to what you eat daily. Be careful with supplements because of the potential for magnesium toxicity and make sure you let your doctor know that you are also on supplements. Why should you consider paying more attention to magnesium than you may have done in the past?

According to the National Institute health, magnesium affects membrane integrity, muscle contraction, hormone secretion and intermediary metabolism. Magnesium also helps in the movement of calcium and potassium across cell membranes, that can affect heart rhythm and nerve conduction. Recent research findings have shown that magnesium can help your brain health by helping your brain shrink less with less white matter lesions. Researchers also found that taking magnesium per day as recommended could lead to less risk of memory loss, age-related dementia, and help one to keep cognitive functions for longer as we get older.

The other two things that you can do that will help protect your brain health and memory will be taking more steps every day and doing more puzzles or doing more activity books weekly. When it comes to puzzles and activity books , do one new book per week.

Another way to stay mentally active and stay connected to a community is to get a hobby. Develop a noteworthy hobby that you can practice with a group of people in a safe environment. This will help you adjust your work-life balance and lessen or minimize the impact of problems in your daily life. Your hobby could be playing baseball, basketball, golf, dancing, fishing, running, tennis or even playing Sudoku. It could also be any other unique activity that preferably has a mental, spiritual and physical component that you can participate in on a regular basis that would help take your mind away from the activities that typically consume your day.

What is your self-care strategy for managing active illness? Do you collaborate with your doctors? Do you listen to them, then ask questions and take action that will help you become better? You need to take your medications, do the tests that you are asked to do and go to your appointments. If still in doubt or need further assurance about the direction of care or your prognosis, seek a second opinion.

If you have not seen your doctor in a long time set up an appointment with your health care provider to enable you get a more detailed picture of your metabolic profile, especially your cholesterol level, blood sugar, potassium, vitamin D and other tests relevant to your family and medical history. Do you have a family or personal history of obesity–related illnesses like diabetes, high blood pressure, heart attack or stroke?

# 8 Keys To Longevity After 50

If you have a blood pressure cuff, measure your blood pressure today. If you do not have one, go to the nearest pharmacy, and use their free blood pressure cuff to find out your blood pressure. The steps outlined so far are things you can do for yourself now, especially if you feel you are healthy but have not taken any objective steps to check your health for years. Maybe your last health check was in school or when you got hired or just before you retired.

What are the other important self-care aspects you need to know and do? Do you brush your teeth every morning and night?

Do you ignore your oral health and personal hygiene in your health and wellness journey? Poor oral health can lead to systemic diseases like heart disease, pneumonia and cancer to name a few.

Do you get your immunizations as needed? If you need to get vaccines, get your vaccines like the flu vaccines or COVID 19 vaccines. Do not just say you are eating healthy, exercising, and taking your

---

supplements; therefore, you do not need to get your vaccines. If you need to bundle up because it is cold, do it. Wash your hands frequently to minimize your chances of getting an infection.

Do you also know that focusing on gratitude despite your daily changes can be part of your daily self-care?

An attitude of gratitude will help you deal with daily challenging situations calmly. This will help you to overcome your stress.

Stay vigilant when you are interacting with others. Stay vigilant during your conversations with others. Be careful about when you speak and be careful about what you speak about. Learn to lower expectations during your interactions with others. Lower the expectation that you will be understood or that your own context or perspective will be understood. This will help to have better emotional balance, which is a very important aspect of your emotional wellness and holistic self-care.

What about sociocultural self-care? Are you a value adding person? Do you add value to your culture and community? As you get older people can say that you have contributed positively to your cultural heritage. Do you stay connected to your community?

What about your spiritual self-care? Do what is right for your spirituality without condemning others? Do you do your meditations and regularly go to your faith-based services. Research shows that if you have a lifestyle with spirituality and religion, you have a healthier and longer life!

Making sure you sleep well is an important part of your holistic self-care. Do you pay attention to your self-care as you get older? Do you know your patterns? What is holding you back from improving your health every day? Is it that you are too busy? Is it that you don't have a better self-mastery of yourself? While self-mastery requires more mental energy to set up, once you have achieved greater self-mastery you will require less energy to function more effectively through good positive healthy habits. Your brain likes to reduce the energy it spends to accomplish tasks, which is part of the reason we form habits. Research has shown that about 40 % to 50% of our daily activities are shaped by habits. Do you know the habits that dominate your own daily activities? Are they good habits or bad habits?

Do you deal with stress by smoking or drinking alcohol? Do you know drinking too much alcohol is not good for your health?

*Don't smoke. If  you are still smoking, make plans to stop. Don't use smoking, alcohol and sex as coping mechanisms for managing stress or dealing with challenging or negative relationships.

Do you know the patterns that dominate your relationships, activities and eating habits?

Do you know how to maintain your positive emotional wellness during your daily interactions with others?

Consider taking advantage of free informational health exams or blood work offered at your office or your membership clubs or insurance to get your cholesterol or metabolic profile. Find out your weight and your height and using both figures with your age calculate your body mass index (BMI). Why is your BMI important? It helps you to find out your likelihood of having heart disease, diabetes, or some cancers. Wow! Wouldn't you like to know the risk for such deadly killers?

*Do you have a family history of high blood pressure, diabetes, cancer, or glaucoma?

*Start each day with meditation and exercise and a plan for the day.

*Keep quiet if you have nothing positive to say.

*Become familiar with your family and medical history.

---

# 8 Keys To Longevity  After  50

*Review your health insurance regularly.

*Get more education. That will help you become a better health self-advocate

*Stay vigilant in all your interactions with others.

*Pain begets pain.

* What area of self -improvement did you focus on in the past 72 hours?

*Continue to write down your emotions periodically.

*Forgive yourself and others daily

*Sleep at least seven to eight hours a day.

*Cut down on unnecessary expenses.

*Call a friend today.

*Review your finances.

---

# 8 Keys To Longevity  After  50

*Do you go for your yearly or biyearly eye checkup?

*How much money do you make in a week and how much money do you spend in a week?

 *What simple steps can you take today to have better health?

*Help at least one person each day.

*Meditate or say a prayer or do both.

*Form a healthy living group of friends and family that you can trust or join one.

*Repeat your blood pressure check.

*Weigh yourself regularly.

*Take your multivitamins regularly.

*Become familiar what the time of the day you deal with most quarrels and conflicts

*Is it at night, day, or morning?

# 8 Keys To Longevity  After  50

*Put in the time to learn more about the things that matter to you.


*Work for your  future everyday
.

*Continue to write on journal at least once a week.
.

After the check up, you have to follow through with the labs and tests you have to do. You have to go to the pharmacy and get your medications. After you get your medications, you must take them or make sure you don't mix them up when taking them, if not you will not get the desired result.

Please keep your goals simple and related to the 8 Keys to longevity that can help you make the healthy lifestyle choices that can help you to live a healthier and longer more fulfilled life.

It is also important to remember that research shows that gratitude has elements of subjective well-being such as lower negative effect, life satisfaction, and higher positive effect and elements of psychosocial or eudaimonic well-being such as purpose in life, personal autonomy, positive relations with others and environmental mastery ( Mills et al, 2015 ).

*You can list 3 things you are grateful for every day.

*Plant gratitude trees for your birthday. You can plant it for every birthday or plant it for your 50th birthday, 60th, 65th birthday, 70th and so on.

*You can start a gratitude journal that you fill out every weekend.

*You can pray for more gratitude if you are a person of faith, or you can meditate on gratitude.

*Challenge yourself to be grateful for people, conditions, and things.

---

*Share your sense of gratitude with others and encourage them to share their own sense of gratitude.

Challenge yourself to form habits that will help you review and improve daily. What is the essence of your holistic wellness and healthy living if it will not help you live a happy, healthy, longer, and more positive and fulfilled life? The decision to live a happier, healthier, and longer life has to be supported by consistent good habits and your own compass blueprint for healthy living.

Make a list of the barriers to your health and longevity program and how you plan to overcome them every day. What changes do you think you can make that will help you to live a healthier and longer life?

What will do every day to review and improve your health and wellness daily? Here are 30 questions you can answer as part of your 30-day holistic self-care challenge.

---

# 8 Keys To Longevity After 50

Here are examples of the few things you can do regularly as part of daily holistic self-care:

*Do you start each day with meditation, exercise and a to-do list?

*Do you keep stress out of your relationship?

*Did you know that cutting down on unnecessary expenses can help you have better financial wellness?

*Did you call a friend today as part of positive and supportive relationships?

*Have helped at least one stranger or someone you didn't know in the past 7 days?

*Write down your feelings and experiences.

# 8 Keys To Longevity  After  50

*Do check your blood pressure once a week or as often as you have been asked to by your doctor?

*Do you weigh yourself every 3 days or at least once a week?

*Do you take your multivitamins or supplements regularly?

*Do you keep your appointment with your healthcare providers?

*When was the last time you failed to stay vigilant in all your interactions with others?

*Do you forgive yourself and others daily?

* How many people did you not forgive last week?

*Write down what time of the day you are in much pain.

*Don't expect others to forgive you because you apologized or explained your perspective.

*How many times a day did you keep quiet when  you had nothing positive to say?

*Do you take a deep breath before you respond to stressful situations.

* What area of self -improvement did you focus on in the past 72 hours?

*How many times did you sleep at least seven to eight hours a day in the past one week?

*How many times did you reach out to a friend or relative in the past one week?

# 8 Keys To Longevity After 50

*How much money do you make in a week and how much money do you spend in a week?

*Cut down on unnecessary expenses.

*What simple steps can you take today to have better health?

*Do you pray every day?

*Have you formed a healthy living group of friends and family that you can trust or joined one?

*Write down your feelings and experiences.

*Do your blood pressure check at least once a week.
How many hours a day do you spend on social media or on the phone?

*Get a blood pressure logbook and use it.

*Keep your appointment with your healthcare providers.

# 8 Keys To Longevity After 50

*Keep eating right even after a lapse.

*When was the last time you did your yearly physical?

*Take care of your oral health, personal hygiene and self-care

*Do you do your screening tests as recommended by your healthcare providers?

*Become familiar with your family and medical history.

*Do you have the most quarrels and conflicts in the morning, afternoon , and evening?

*Have you reviewed your health insurance in the past 30 days?

*Do you put in the time to learn more about the things that are good for your health?

*Do you protect your home from falls and accidents?

# 8 Keys To Longevity After 50

*Work for your future everyday

.

*Do you write down your emotional challenges every 3 days?

*Do you say 3 things you are grateful for every day?

.

*Stick to daily supportive communications.

*How many hours do you spend watching TV every day?

*Do you drink alcohol to cope with stress or your daily challenges?

*Do you like to get things done step by step or on the fly?

Start your own longevity journal. Start a health and wellness journal. Get pen and paper and write down your own answers to the questions above or type them into your computer, phone, or mobile device. Do some journaling to keep tabs on yourself. Begin by setting realistic health and wellness goals for yourself.

What is your 30-day  holistic self-care challenge? What percentage of your time in the past 7 days did you put into doing the things that could help you improve your holistic self-care? The answers you give to these questions will help find out if you are doing your best to improve your holistic self-care at least 80% of the time. Keeping to the 80:20 rule through your habits, daily activities, and lifestyle changes will help begin to live a healthier, happier, longer and more fulfilled life as you get older!

## Notes

Ardell DB(1999), Definition of wellness. Ardell Wellness Report,1999, 1-5.

Bains P (2020) Exercise to live longer. Allina Health

Be well BU; Learn practices that lead to better health and well-being. www.belmont.edu

Bussing A, Wirth AG, Reiser F, Zahn A, Humbroich K, Gerbersghagen K, Baumann K. Experience of gratitude, awe and beauty in life among patients with multiple sclerosis and psychiatric disorders. Health Qual Life outcomes.2014;12:63. https://pubmed.ncbi.nim.nih.gov/25102199/

CDC.gov; LDL and HDL Cholesterol: "Bad" and "Good" Cholesterol

Crouch M(2019) AARP

Chung I, (2005)Stress-Induced Atherosclerosis: Clinical Evidence and Possible Underlying Mechanism, Korean Circulation J 2005;35:101-105
Microsoft Word - 슌2-1.doc (koreamed.org)


Debbie L Stoewen, ( 2017) Dimensions of Wellness. Can Vet J, 58(8): 861-862

Healing yourself with self-hypnosis, Frank Caprio, M.D. and joseph R Berger

Lin, J. and Epel, E.(2022) Stress and telomere shortening; Insights from cellular mechanisms. Ageing Res Rev.2022 Jan:73:101507. Published online 2021 Nov 1.doi 10.1016/j.arr.2021.101507

Mels Carbonell, Ph.D., How to solve the people puzzle. Uniquely You Resources, 2008.

Mills PJ, Redwine L, Wilson K, Pung MA, Chinh K, Greenberg BH, Lunde O, Maisel A, Raisinghani A, Wood A, Chopra D. The

Role of Gratitude in Spiritual Well-being in Asymptomatic Heart Failure Patients. Spiritual Clin Pract (Wash D C ). 2015 Mar;2(1):5-17. doi: 10.1037/scp0000050. PMID: 26203459; PMCID: PMC4507265.

National Council on Aging(NCOA).(2023), Get the facts on Healthy Aging. www.ncoa.org

National Institutes of Health(.gov) https://www.ncbi.nih.gov.pmc
NSC(National Safety Council)2023: Injury Facts: Deaths by Demographics: Top 10 Preventable Injuries
https://injuryfacts.nsc.org//all-in

National Institute of Health(NIH) News.(2017), You're Never too Old. Keep active as you age.
https;//newsinhealth.nih.gov/special-issues/seniors/youre-never-too-old

Poljšak B, Milisav I. Clinical implications of cellular stress responses. Bosn J Basic Med Sci. 2012 May;12(2):122-6. doi:

10.17305/bjbms.2012.2510.          PMID: 22642596; PMCID: PMC4362434

Robin G. Better Than Before: Mastering the Habits of Our Everyday Lives.Toronto, Ontario, Pengium Random House, Doubleday Canada, 2015.

Renna, M.E.(2021) A review and novel theoretical model of how negative emotions influence inflammation: The critical role of emotion regulation. Brain Behav Immun Health. 2021,Nov 25. Doi:10.1016/j.bbih.2021.100397 Retrieved from https://www.ncbi.nlm.nih.gov/pmc/articles/PMC8649080/

Sabot D, Lovegrove R, Stapleton P. The association between sleep quality and telomere length: A systematic literature review. Brain Behav Immun Health. 2023 Jan 9;28:100577. doi: 10.1016/j.bbih.2022.100577. PMID: 36691437; PMCID: PMC9860369.

---

Salleh MR. Life event, stress and illness. Malays J Med Sci. 2008 Oct;15(4):9-18. PMID: 22589633; PMCID: PMC3341916.

Shammas MA. Telomeres, lifestyle, cancer, and aging. Curr Opin Clin Nutr Metab Care. 2011 Jan;14(1):28-34. doi: 10.1097/MCO.0b013e32834121b1. PMID: 21102320; PMCID: PMC3370421.
Sorriento D, Di Vaia E, Iaccarino G. Physical Exercise: A Novel Tool to Protect Mitochondrial Health. Front Physiol. 2021 Apr 27;12:660068. doi: 10.3389/fphys.2021.660068. PMID: 33986694; PMCID: PMC8110831.

Smith, K. S., & Graybiel, A. M. (2016). Habit formation. *Dialogues in clinical neuroscience, 18*(1), 33–43. https://doi.org/10.31887/DCNS.2016.18.1/ksmith
Retrieved from Habit formation (nih.gov)

University of New Hamshire2023, Health & Wellness. www.unh.edu
https://www.unh.edu/health/intellectual wellness

---

University of Maryland:Dimensions of Wellness. Retrieved from (last accessed 2021) https://www.umaryland.edu/wellness/dimensions-of-wellness

Wood AM, Maltby J. Stewart N, Linley PA, Joseph S.(2008). A social-cognitive model of trait and state levels of gratitude. Emotion,2008;8(2):281-280. https://pubmed.ncbi.nim.nih.gov [Google Scholar]

WHO (2020)The top ten causes of death https://www.who.int/news-room/fact-sheets/details/the-top-10-causes-of-death

Yaribeygi H, Panahi Y, Sahraei H, Johnston TP, Sahebkar A. The impact of stress on body function: A review. EXCLI J. 2017 Jul 21;16:1057-1072. doi: 10.17179/excli2017-480. PMID: 28900385; PMCID: PMC5579396.

## Resources

Here are additional resources that will help you live a healthier and longer life by consistently trying to be the best version of yourself in all aspects of your life. Did you know that you can become the best and happiest version of yourself every day irrespective of the situation or circumstance you may  find yourself in?

www.compasswellnessinstitute.com

http://www.amazon.com/Dr.-Chio-Ugochukwu/e/B00JNFLPQQ

Join the compass club on Facebook

https://www.facebook.com/groups/1748276835431116/

**Other books by Dr. Chio Ugochukwu that will help you improve your health, eliminate stress and transform your life include;**

**The Compass Health Transformer: Your 72 Hour Blue Print For Healthy Living**

In this book you will learn more about how doing the 72-hour food audit can help

---

you gain a better understanding of how you can improve your health through easy daily adjustments …..

## 21 Ways To Transform Your Health Without Medications

"…21 simple proven ways to reduce stress and improve your health and wellbeing without relying on medications. These are easy and effective ways you can use to turn your daily challenges into transformative opportunities for healthy living and daily happiness. You can start right away without spending a fortune!.."

**<u>Get your own copy of 21 Ways To Transform Your Health Without Medications</u>**

**Overcoming Daily Stress: 21 Quick And Easy Ways To Stay Stress-Free In Your Daily Life**

"…Are you tired of being stressed out everyday? Are you tired of feeling exhausted and overwhelmed in your daily activities? Are you fed up with communication issues in your relationship? Here are 21 quick and easy ways you can use to overcome daily stress and turn your daily challenges into opportunities for transformative abundant living. This book will help you gain a better understanding of your potential communication issues, daily 'stress points' and the steps you can take to overcome them…".

## Get your own copy of Overcoming Daily Stress

## The Secret To Daily happiness

 "..Have you ever wondered why daily happiness has continued to elude you? Do you want to make sustainable daily happiness part of your life? By reading this book
you can find answers to these questions and many more on how to overcome the many obstacles and challenges that daily try to take away your inner peace and contentment…"

## <u>Get your own copy of The Secret To Happiness</u>

## 15 Simple Ways to lower your blood pressure naturally after 40 without complicated diets

"……Don't spend your most productive years dealing with high blood pressure, medications and side effects. Stop worrying about whether you forgot to take your first medication or the second one. Take these simple steps to lower your blood pressure naturally and minimize your need for multiple medications. Did you know that high blood pressure can cause heart attacks, stroke, kidney failure, blindness and memory problems? Don't wait to find out! Take Action! ,,,,,"

<u>Click Here for Your own copy of 15 Simple Ways To Reduce Blood Pressure....</u>

Here is a book to help lose fat. If your main concern or focus is losing pounds you have accumulated as fat then get a copy of the book

---

## "How To Lose 23 Pounds of Fat Without Torture Diets or Hard Exercise And keep it (The Compass Method).

"Are you fed up with trying to lose weight again and again with limited success? Are you tired of all the confusing new and expensive diets you have tried to follow every day with zero results? Do you want the health benefits of living with optimum weight without following complicated rules? Do you want to become more energetic and active again? Are you fed up with the wild ride of losing weight today and gaining it back tomorrow? Then read this book so that you will start using a comprehensive individualized weight loss strategy that will help you lose fat and keep it off, without going on torture diets or deadly strenuous exercises. You will learn to do this through the Compass Method that is based on a holistic approach to weight-loss, healthy living and personal transformation."

If prayer is something that appeals to you, you might be interested in the following next two books that incorporate prayers into our daily strive to become better and become more fulfilled:

**Praying To Win: How To Get More Victories And Riches In Your Daily Life Through Spiritual Principles**

"..You too can achieve your goals and dreams, through praying to win. You can do this by immersing yourself in the word of God and transforming the moments that make up your daily life through persistent adoration……. Above all, thank God every day, never give up and persistently continue praying to win…"

Get your own copy of Praying To Win

**9 Best Ways To Eliminate Stress, Improve Your Health And thrive Without Limitations Through Prayers**

Are tired of being knocked down by stress from your daily hassles? Are you tired of dealing with chronic illnesses associated with stress? Do you want to live a fun-filled daily life? Here are 9 of the best ways you can change your daily obstacles and challenges into opportunities to thrive without limitations through the power of prayers.

## Too Young To Die

"A book about coping with grief and finding your way in life…"

## 9 Best Ways To Quit Smoking Without Becoming A Nervous Wreck And Gaining Weight

"..Here are 9 of the best ways to finally quit smoking without becoming a nervous wreck or gaining weight. If you have tried to quit smoking before, but failed or tried to quit but was overcome by anxiety or fear of becoming socially awkward or gaining weight, then read this book! This book was previously published as "The Compass Health Transformer Quit Smoking" but has been rewritten to include the transtheoretical model of change to help you get a better understanding of where you are in your journey or process of quitting smoking. The

9 best ways to quit smoking also includes a reminder of the different ways smoking can affect your health and body and the different individualized-changes you can make to your life-style to help you quit smoking on your own terms.

## 9 Best Ways To Deal With Negative People, Protect Your Health And Be Happy

"..Are you tired of being stressed out by encounters with negative people? Are you fed up with the impact of negative situations on your health and happiness? Would like you to find out ways to remain effective during negative situations and encounters with negative people? Do you know that chronic stress generated by negative encounters can damage your eyes, heart and brain? Do you know that chronic stress can directly damage your body cells? Here are 9 best ways you can protect your health from such negative situations so that you can continue to thrive and be happy..".

**To order new or additional copies or ask questions, please visit:**

http://www.amazon.com/Dr.-Chio-Ugochukwu/e/B00JNFLPQQ

Call or Text : 661 992 6436

Join the Compass club @

https://www.facebook.com/compassclub

## About the Author

Dr. Chio Ugochukwu has always been interested in helping people improve their health and wellness, and live a healthier, longer and more fulfilled life through simple habits and strategies and for better self-care. He is focused on helping individuals and groups, develop their own compass blueprint for healthy living, and self-mastery. Doing the 30-day challenge in this book will help you learn how to stay more consistently physically active, sleep better, become more efficient at managing stress, and chronic conditions, and have more positive and supportive relationships.

Dr. Chio was inspired to develop the compass method for transformational living, through the challenges he has encountered in his journey of life, his practice of medicine, and his fascination with how the mind, the spirit and human experience influence the accomplishment of goals and the fulfillment of life, and his ancient heritage of Ozaa Akwusina (Warriors Never Stop).

He is the medical director of the Compass Wellness Institute and a consultant and specialist with interests in integrative medicine, ophthalmology, medical informatics, and public health. As an author, researcher, and consultant, he has peer reviewed publications on health and quality of life, and published more than 100 books and articles, on health and wellness, eye health, weight management, conflict management, stress management, effective communication, and integrative self-mastery habits.

To get some of Dr. Chio's books please visit:
https://www.amazon.com/author/chio